LIBRARY

Learning
Resource Centre

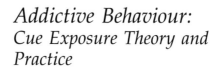

Addictive Behaviour:
Cue Exposure Theory and
Practice

THE WILEY SERIES IN CLINICAL PSYCHOLOGY

Series Editor
J. Mark G. Williams *Department of Psychology, University College of North Wales, Bangor, UK*

D. Colin Drummond, Stephen T. Tiffany, Steven Glautier and Bob Remington (Editors)	Addictive Behaviour: Cue Exposure Theory and Practice
Carlo Perris, Willem A. Arrindell and Martin Eisemann (Editors)	Parenting and Psychopathology
Chris Barker, Nancy Pistrang and Robert Elliott	Research Methods in Clinical and Counselling Psychology
Graham C.L. Davey and Frank Tallis (Editors)	Worrying: Perspectives on Theory, Assessment and Treatment
Paul Dickens	Quality and Excellence in Human Services

Further titles in preparation

A list of earlier titles in the series follows the index

Edited by

D. COLIN
DRUMMOND
STEPHEN T.
TIFFANY
STEVEN GLAUTIER
BOB REMINGTON

Addictive Behaviour:
Cue Exposure Theory
and Practice

With a Foreword by

G. ALAN
MARLATT

JOHN WILEY & SONS

Chichester · New York · Brisbane · Toronto · Singapore

Copyright © 1995 by   John Wiley & Sons Ltd,
                       Baffins Lane, Chichester,
                       West Sussex PO19 1UD, England

                       National   01243 779777
                       International   (+44) 1243 779777

Reprinted December 1995

Other Wiley Editorial Offices

John Wiley & Sons, Inc., 605 Third Avenue,
New York, NY 10158-0012, USA

Jacaranda Wiley Ltd, 33 Park Road, Milton,
Queensland 4064, Australia

John Wiley & Sons (Canada) Ltd, 22 Worcester Road,
Rexdale, Ontario M9W 1L1, Canada

John Wiley & Sons (SEA) Pte Ltd, 37 Jalan Pemimpin #05-04,
Block B, Union Industrial Building, Singapore 2057

Library of Congress Cataloging-in-Publication Data

Addictive behaviour: cue exposure theory and practice / edited by D. Colin
    Drummond . . . [et al.].
        p.   cm. — (The Wiley series in clinical psychology)
    Includes bibliographical references and indexes.
    ISBN 0-471-94454-8 (cased)
    1. Substance abuse.   I. Drummond, D. Colin.   II. Series.
    [DNLM: 1. Substance Dependence—psychology.   2. Substance
    Dependence — therapy.   3. Behavior, Addictive.   4. Cues.   WM 270
    A22463 1995]
    RC564.A323   1995
    616.86—dc20
    DNLM/DLC
    for Library of Congress   94–23956
                                                                    CIP

British Library Cataloguing in Publication Data

A catalogue record for this book is available from the British Library

ISBN 0-471-94454-8

Typeset in 10/12 pt Palatino by Photo·graphics, Honiton, Devon
Printed and bound in Great Britain by Bookcraft (Bath) Ltd
This book is printed on acid-free paper responsibly manufactured from sustainable
forestation, for which at least two trees are planted for each one used for paper
production.

CONTENTS

ABOUT THE EDITORS

D. Colin Drummond   *Division of Addictive Behaviour, 6th Floor, Hunter Wing, St George's Hospital Medical School, University of London, Cranmer Terrace, London SW17 0RE, UK*

Stephen T. Tiffany   *Department of Psychological Sciences, Purdue University, 1364 Psychological Sciences Building, West Lafayette, Indiana 47907-1364, USA*

Steven Glautier   *Centre for Substance Abuse Research, Department of Psychology, University of Wales Swansea, SA2 8PP, UK*

Bob Remington   *Department of Psychology, University of Southampton, Highfield, Southampton SO9 5NH, UK*

Colin Drummond is a Senior Lecturer in Addictive Behaviour and Honorary Consultant Psychiatrist in the Division of Addictive Behaviour, St George's Hospital Medical School, University of London, UK. He previously worked in the Addiction Research Unit, National Addiction Centre, Institute of Psychiatry, University of London. Dr Drummond studied medicine at the University of Glasgow, and his research thesis is entitled "Alcohol Related Problems and Public Health". He is a member of the Royal College of Psychiatrists and the Society for the Study of Addiction, and is assistant editor of the journal *Addiction*. He has conducted a wide range of research studies in the addictions field and is responsible for the development of community-based treatment services for problem drinkers in London. Amongst his research publications are several studies in cue exposure in alcohol dependence.

Stephen Tiffany is a Professor of Psychology at Purdue University in West Lafayette, Indiana. He received his PhD in clinical psychology from the

University of Wisconsin-Madison and completed a clinical internship in the Department of Psychiatry at the University of Wisconsin-Madison. He has conducted extensive human and animal research on addictive disorders and has authored over 40 professional publications. In 1993 he received the American Psychological Association Distinguished Scientific Award for Early Career Contribution to Psychology.

Steven Glautier is a Lecturer in Psychology working in the Department of Psychology at the University of Wales, Swansea. His PhD, from Southampton University, was on classical conditioning in human subjects using alcohol as a reinforcer and was obtained whilst he was working in London at the Institute of Psychiatry's Addiction Research Unit. His main research interest is in the application of principles of learning and behaviour to addiction. He is currently an assistant editor for the journal *Addiction* and a member of the British Psychological Society.

Bob Remington is Professor of Psychology and Head of Department at the University of Southampton. All his research has been concerned with issues arising from an analysis of the role of basic learning processes in human behaviour. Some of this work has been of direct theoretical interest, e.g. conditioning and habituation processes, while other aspects have focused on the practical application of learning principles in clinical, social and educational contexts. His previous book, *The Challenge of Severe Mental Handicap: A Behaviour Analytic Approach*, is also published by Wiley.

LIST OF CONTRIBUTORS

David B. Abrams   *Division of Behavioural Medicine, Brown University School of Medicine and The Miriam Hospital, 164 Summit Avenue, Providence, RI 02906, USA*

Timothy B. Baker   *Center for Tobacco Research and Intervention, University of Wisconsin Medical School, 1300 University Avenue, Madison, Wisconsin 53706, USA*

Thomas H. Brandon   *Department of Psychology, State University of New York at Binghamton, PO Box 6000, Binghamton, New York 13902-6000, USA*

Sharon Dawe   *National Drug and Alcohol Research Centre, University of New South Wales, PO Box 1, Kensington, Sydney, New South Wales 2033, Australia*

Janet Greeley   *Department of Psychology and Sociology, James Cook University, Townsville, Queensland 4811, Australia*

Nick Heather   *Northern Regional Alcohol and Drug Service, Plummer Court, Carliol Place, Newcastle-upon-Tyne NE1 6UR, UK*

Peter M. Monti   *Veterans Affairs Medical Center, and Center for Alcohol and Addiction Studies, Brown University, Box G-BH, Providence, RI 02912, USA*

Thomas M. Piasecki   *Center for Tobacco Research and Intervention, University of Wisconsin Medical School, 1300 University Avenue, Madison, Wisconsin 53706, USA*

Jane H. Powell   *Psychology Department, Goldsmiths College, University of London, New Cross, London SE14 6NW, UK*

Edward P. Quinn — *Department of Psychology, State University of New York at Binghamton, PO Box 6000, Binghamton, New York 13902-6000, USA*

Vaughan W. Rees — *National Drug and Alcohol Research Centre, University of New South Wales, PO Box 1, Kensington, Sydney, New South Wales 2033, Australia*

Damaris J. Rohsenow — *Veterans Affairs Medical Center, and Center for Alcohol and Addiction Studies, Brown University, Box G-BH, Providence, RI 02912, USA*

Colin Ryan — *Department of Psychology and Sociology, James Cook University, Townsville, Queensland 4811, Australia*

FOREWORD

My first exposure to the topic of this book occurred during my internship in clinical psychology at Napa State Hospital in California. It was the late 1960s, at the height of the hippie era in nearby San Francisco. I was assigned to work with a patient on the inpatient alcoholism-treatment ward. The patient was a man in his early thirties, a single, blue-collar worker who lived alone in a small apartment in the rundown Tenderloin district of the city prior to his admission to the hospital for alcohol detox-ification and treatment. My supervisor, a psychologist critical of the Twelve-Step disease model treatment program used on the ward, advised me to take a different approach: insight-oriented psychotherapy (his own specialty). Over the month-long inpatient program, I met with the patient twice a week for hour-long therapy sessions, exploring vari-ous potential determinants of his drinking problem, with an emphasis on exploring and developing insight into early childhood abuse from his alcoholic father and various other traumas. As the sessions progressed, the patient appeared to gain more and more insight into the roots of his alcohol dependence. As the day of his discharge arrived, he was keenly optimistic about his chances for recovery. "Don't worry, Dr Marlatt," I recall him saying that Friday morning as he left to board the Greyhound Bus bound for San Francisco, "I now know why I became an alcoholic and why I should never take another drink in my life!" I even confessed to my supervisor that insight therapy seemed to be working and was eager to support his attempts to make this form of treatment more avail-able on the alcoholism unit.

Our optimism was short lived. My patient was readmitted to the detox unit Monday morning after a severe weekend binge. When he was back on his feet a few days later, I asked him what had happened. "It all happened so fast, I wasn't prepared for it!" he said, explaining that the bus had dropped him off right in front of a bar in the Tenderloin district Friday at noon. Seeing the bar's neon lights and the open door, he wand-ered in as if pulled by a magnet. "I couldn't stop myself from drinking once I was in the bar," he told me, adding: "Dr Marlatt, you helped me see WHY I became an alcoholic and WHY I should never drink again, but you said nothing much about HOW exactly I was supposed to do it!"

It struck me then how right he was. As a clinical psychologist trained in a behavioral psychology department of the "Dustbowl Empiricism", tradition in the American midwest, how could I overlook the obvious? Here was a patient with a severe behavioral problem: excessive drinking. At Indiana University, I studied conditioning theory and worked in the labs of such mentors as Professors Isadore Gormezano and John Ost (classical conditioning with rabbits and dogs, respectively) and James Dinsmoor (operant conditioning with pigeons). As clinical students, we were steeped in learning and reinforcement theory. My first publication was in the area of human eyelid conditioning and my dissertation consisted of a verbal conditioning study. Behavior therapy was then in its infancy with its foundations firmly established in conditioning theory.

I examined the alcoholism treatment program at Napa through the eyes of a budding behavior therapist. As someone steeped in stimulus-response theory as a basis for behavioral interventions, the most obvious question was: Where is the stimulus? If drinking is the target behavior, why is the patient treated in the complete absence of any alcohol cues or drinking contexts? Early behavioral theorists based in Hullian learning theory had already postulated drive-reduction as a reinforcer for alcohol consumption in animals and humans in the form of the tension–reduction hypothesis. Operant labs began in the late sixties to study the drinking behavior of alcoholics in controlled ward settings, pioneered by the work of Peter Nathan, Nancy Mello, Jack Mendelsohn, and others. None of this work appeared to have any impact on the alcoholism treatment program at Napa State.

Instead of exposing patients to drinking/drug cues in an attempt to prepare them for the inevitable temptations of the real-world environment, every attempt was made to remove all such stimuli from the inpatient treatment context. There were no alcoholic beverages (real or in photographic format) to be seen, no bar, no alcohol ads, not even a single shot glass. It was as if the goal of the treatment program was to keep patients behind a protective shield, screened from all temptations to drink, all fruits forbidden. The only time patients were allowed to even mention drinking or alcohol was in "Drunkalogue" confessions during AA meetings, and there the emphasis was usually on the evils of drink. Was it any surprise, therefore, that patients such as the one I worked with were totally unprepared for the naturalistic alcohol cue exposure they experienced shortly after discharge from the program?

These early internship experiences have had a lasting impact on my own professional career interests in the addictive behaviors field. I began by developing treatment interventions in which alcohol cues played a key role. During my years at the University of Wisconsin in the early 1970s, I built my first experimental bar in the basement of the alcoholism treatment building at Mendota State Hospital. The bar was used to provide a realistic drinking context for patients who were treated with electrical aversion therapy. Assessment of the environmental context of relapse for these patients led to the development of relapse prevention programs to help prepare patients to cope with high-risk situations that might otherwise trigger a return to drinking. In my current position at the University of Washington, we have conducted much of our human drinking research in a simulated tavern called BARLAB (Behavioral Alcohol Research Laboratory)—a setting that mimics the cues of a natural drinking setting.

All of which brings me to say why I am so enthusiastic about this book, the first comprehensive coverage of cue exposure in the addictive behavior field to appear within a single volume! Much has happened in this area of research since I treated my first patient with alcohol problems over twenty-five years ago (if only this book were available then!). As noted in the preface, senior editors Colin Drummond (British) and Stephen Tiffany (American), hatched the idea for putting this book together at the 1991 meeting of the Research Society on Alcoholism. The product of this transatlantic cooperation is truly worthy of praise, and I applaud their efforts along with that of their junior editors, Steven Glautier and Bob Remington. The editors have brought together an impressive international list of authors to the table, a literal "Who's Who" of cue exposure experts drawn from the USA, the UK, and Australia. The book spans three main areas of interest: theoretical models of cue exposure (Chapters 2 and 3), methods to study human drug cue reactivity (Chapters 4, 5, 6, and 7), and the clinical application of cue exposure in the treatment of addictive behaviors (Chapters 8, 9, and 10). There is a great deal in this smorgasbord of chapters to whet the appetite of many readers. I think the material would be of particular interest to both academics and scientist–practitioners. There is much rich theoretical discussion to satisfy the appetites of most academics and researchers, especially those with a background and interest in conditioning and learning (including cognitive and social learning). Graduate students in clinical and health psychology, behavioral medicine, psychopharmacology, public health, as well as medical students and interns, will benefit from the breadth and depth of the coverage. Those working as practitioners, helping clients with dependence problems with alcohol, opiates, cocaine and nicotine, will find a variety of tempting offerings, particularly in the three final chapters. Basic research scientists will appreciate the detail in describing methods to assess cue reactivity in a variety of subject populations.

Despite the many advances documented in the present volume, there is still resistance to accepting and implementing cue exposure methods in alcohol and substance abuse treatment. In one recent survey of alcohol and drug counselors, cue exposure and aversion therapy were listed as potentially harmful treatment procedures. Part of this problem can be traced to ignorance about the values of cue exposure in clinical practice (e.g. as a method to assess degree of dependence by measuring cue reactivity across several response domains). Another factor contributing to this resistance is the failure of passive cue-exposure programs to lead to a lasting extinction of reactivity outside the immediate treatment environment. Recent programs that combine cue exposure with active coping skill training for relapse prevention (as described in Chapter 8, for example) appear more promising in terms of post-treatment outcomes. As one modality in a comprehensive behavioral treatment program, cue exposure offers considerable promise for both assessment and intervention.

One sometimes forgets how important cue exposure theory and practice is for our clients in treatment (and for those of us who attempt to change our own habit patterns). In relapse prevention, we often use a relapse debriefing procedure to help clients understand their own relapse chains and high-risk cues. This is especially helpful for those who attribute their setbacks to internal factors beyond their control—such as an addictive disease, genetics, or lack of internal willpower. Such clients are usually relieved of their sense of helplessness or guilt when they realize that their urge or lapse may have been triggered by an external cue or situational context. The range of cues that may serve as triggers is potentially infinite (as noted in Chapter 1), including exteroceptive stimuli (the sight, smell and taste of the substance) interoceptive cues (physical drug effects, moods, and cognitions), and withdrawal-related cues. Identification of cues that trigger urges, cravings, and lapses gives the client a handle on the problem—something can be modified or changed.

Just understanding the process of conditioning is helpful to many clients. In this instance I am reminded of another patient I treated at Napa State Hospital in 1968; this one following the first patient whose relapse taught me so much. Based on my prior experience, I was trying to teach this young man (also from the Bay Area) about cues that might precipitate a return to drinking once he left the hospital program. In our final meeting before his discharge was planned, he told me that he had experienced few if any urges to drink in the hospital setting (the policy prohibiting any drinking cues in the treatment environment was still in effect). He told me he felt confident that alcohol would no longer be a problem in his life—he was strongly committed to lifelong abstinence. Without saying anything, I reached down into my briefcase and place a full bottle of Jim Beam bourbon (his favorite) on the desk between us. He looked at the bottle, squirmed in his seat, and tentatively reached for it. Embarrassed, he hesitated, withdrew his hand, and sighed. Clearly just the sight of the bottle severely undermined his resolve. "Maybe I'm not yet ready for discharge," he said, after a long pause. "I had no idea how strong the pull would be. I feel like the dog you told me about the other day, Pavlov's dog who drooled at the sound of the bell! The Jim Beam bottle is my bourbon bell and I need to find a better way to handle it."

The material presented in this book is worth talking about, both with our colleagues and clients alike. This book presents ground-breaking advances in furthering our understanding about the nature of addictive behavior and how to facilitate change in both prevention and treatment arenas. The editors and authors are to be commended for setting such high standards.

G. Alan Marlatt
University of Washington

SERIES PREFACE

There is no dispute about the importance of drug addiction as posing major clinical and social problems. The application of psychological theory to the problem of addictive behaviour has a long history, and of all theories, those relating to cue exposure hold some of the greatest promise. These theories start from the often-made observation that those who have become addicted to a substance find it difficult if they come into contact with anything associated with it. As Drummond and his colleagues point out in their introductory chapter, clinical writing at least as far back as the eighteenth century includes reference to the importance of preventing such exposure. They quote a writer in 1789 who instructed *"Taste not, handle not, touch not* should be inscribed on every vessel that contains spirits in the house of a man who wishes to be cured of the habits of intemperance"*. Can this observation be refined sufficiently to help us understand the underlying processes? How does exposure to such cues lead to craving, and should we distinguish between automatic and non-automatic aspects of such processes? Why do some individuals react more strongly than others to the same cues, and do such differences result in differences in drug-seeking behaviour? Methods for answering these questions, and the implications of these answers for treatment of addictions is the topic of this book. The book makes an important contribution to the addiction literature by building bridges between basic psychological science and clinical practice. It will be valued not only by experimental and clinical psychiatrists and psychologists interested in addiction, but also by students of the subject who wish to find new directions for understanding and treating addictive behaviour.

J. Mark G. Williams
Series Editor

PREFACE

The initial discussion that fertilized the idea of writing this book took place on a sun-drenched beach in Florida: a rare occurrence in academic life, but one which can be highly recommended! The occasion was the annual meeting of the Research Society on Alcoholism in May 1991, and the conversation on that hot afternoon was between two of this book's editors (C.D. and S.T.). We had just contributed to a symposium on cue exposure in alcohol dependence, and as the conversation developed, the need for this book became increasingly apparent. The previous decade had seen a huge increase in published research in cue exposure in the addiction field, from basic science to clinical research. What was clear, however, was that there was a need to take stock of the developments and to take a broader look at where cue exposure was heading. Particularly, there seemed to have been a failure to apply the advances in basic research to the clinical arena in cue exposure. The time was right for a synthesis of the diverse literature on the subject. While there had been many journal publications and isolated book chapters on cue exposure in addictive behaviour, we were not aware of any comprehensive source to which the basic or clinician scientist could refer.

As with so many brief encounters in idyllic far away places, it was not until many months later on a dreary winter London day in December 1991, at the end of another drug cue exposure symposium, this time at the British Psychological Society's London conference, that thoughts once more returned to the conversation on that humid Florida afternoon. A small group of colleagues then came together as an editorial group to discuss the way in which a book on cue exposure in addictive behaviour could best progress. It was agreed at the outset that the book should not end up as a disparate collection of conference papers without a coherent direction or goal. Rather, we decided to commission a series of reviews of the key developing areas of the field and to provide directions for each contributor as to the required scope and coverage. We identified for each contributor the place of each review in the context of the overall direction of the book. In view of the wide array of basic and clinical scientists around the world engaged in addiction cue exposure research, we felt it essential to represent this international mix amongst the contributors. We also deliberately aimed to provide a cross-substance perspective. What was most encouraging was the willingness with which those approached agreed to join the project. They readily identified with the need for and timeliness of the book.

Addictions are responsible for vast and steadily growing morbidity, mortality, and misery in society. Until now the theoretical underpinning of most commonly practised treatment approaches in the addictions field has been scant, and the evidence for the effectiveness of these methods generally lacking. In the cue exposure paradigm there is a rare opportunity to make a vital connection between theory and practice in the rational development of new treatment approaches. However, there is a danger that new approaches become adopted into routine practice in an uncritical fashion. This book therefore aims to provide a much needed critical analysis of the evidence. A further aim of the book is to sensitize basic science researchers, primarily those working with non-human subjects, to the kinds of behaviours that can be modelled in the laboratory. Similarly, there is a need to bring greater awareness of the relevant basic research to those working in the clinical world. This book purposely places itself at the intersection between these diverse and often poorly connected research areas. Finally, the book aims to stimulate interest in the development of further basic and clinical research into cue exposure. Together, the reviews provide a rich source of ideas for future directions that such research could follow.

This book is not a treatment manual that describes how to conduct cue exposure treatment. Rather, it is targeted at basic and clinical scientists in the addictions field. We intend the audience to be principally experimental and clinical psychologists and psychiatrists interested in addiction, but we also intend that the book will appeal to university departments of psychology and psychiatry, to staff, undergraduates and postgraduates, as a teaching and reference text.

The project has come a long way since that germ of an idea came into being on a Florida beach. There has been much discussion, refinement, and (helpful) editorial intervention! The result, we feel, is a detailed but preliminary map of the field of drug cue exposure that will provide much needed impetus and direction for further development.

Our thanks are due to Mike Coombs and Wendy Hudlass of John Wiley & Sons for their support throughout the development of the book; to Griffith Edwards for his comments on the book outline, and for his support of cue exposure research at the Addiction Research Unit, Institute of Psychiatry, over the years. Mandy Holmes provided sterling secretarial support. Finally, we thank our families, Rosaleen and Iona, Kristine and Patrick, Nickey and Ivan, Marina, Becky and Tom, for their patience and constant encouragement.

DCD
STT
SG
BR

CHAPTER 1   Cue exposure in understanding and treating addictive behaviours

D. Colin Drummond*, Stephen T. Tiffany†, Steven Glautier‡ and Bob Remington§

Addiction is the source of extensive and costly problems in society. There is a pressing need for the development of new and more effective treatment approaches in the addictions, and in particular those which have a firm scientific basis. Cue exposure has become a method of key importance in the treatment of phobic and obsessive compulsive disorders. While the effectiveness of cue exposure remains to be conclusively demonstrated in the addictions field, it provides a scientifically based method which shows great promise in advancing our understanding.

Relapse is a common occurrence following a successful period of abstinence from addictive drug use and therefore represents a clinically important phenomenon. Relapse only occurs, by definition, in the presence of the drug, and often takes place when the individual encounters other cues which have been previously associated with drug use. Fortunately, however, relapse is not inevitable. The observation that individuals respond differently to the same set of drug cues provides rich material for the investigation of the causes of relapse and methods to prevent its occurrence.

This chapter describes the development of cue exposure as a method to understand and treat addictive behaviours. We begin by describing different meanings of the term "cue exposure" as applied to addictive behaviours, and proceed to chart the history of its development as a treatment approach. The relationship between cue exposure and other

*St George's Hospital Medical School, University of London, UK, †Purdue University, USA ‡University of Wales, Swansea, UK, and §University of Southampton, UK

Addictive Behaviour: Cue Exposure Theory and Practice.
Edited by D.C. Drummond, S.T. Tiffany, S. Glautier and B. Remington.
© 1995 John Wiley & Sons Ltd.

leading concepts in the addictions is then examined, followed by a résumé of the current status of cue exposure research. Throughout we emphasize the importance of making a connection between basic and clinical science in the rational development of new treatment technologies. Further, we stress that the cue exposure paradigm serves to enhance, rather than compete with, leading theoretical and clinical models of addictive behaviour.

WHAT IS CUE EXPOSURE?

The term "cue exposure" has a number of different meanings. At its most basic, cue exposure refers to a general process in classical conditioning theory. A cue (or stimulus) is presented to an animal, and the response which the animal makes to the cue is dependent on the previous experience that the animal has had with the cue. A cue that has been repeatedly paired with, say, heroin administration can be viewed as a conditioned stimulus (CS) which, when the animal is exposed to the cue alone, can elicit a conditioned response (CR). The more often the cue has been paired with heroin, the greater the likelihood of occurrence and strength of the CR when the animal is exposed to the cue alone. It is also proposed that exposure to a drug cue can, in turn, lead to an increased likelihood of drug self-administration.

It would be wrong, however, to restrict the definition of cue exposure exclusively to a conditioning theory-based mechanism. There are many other possible explanations for the effects of exposure to cues, with social learning theory as a leading alternative candidate. It is true that classical conditioning has been the predominant discourse in cue exposure research in the addictions. However, what is crucially important in the application of cue exposure in the addictions field is that reactivity to drug cues has been repeatedly observed in both animals and humans. The scientific challenge is to explain cue reactivity phenomena. We argue that one does not need to "buy into" classical conditioning theory or, indeed, any other specific theory to study cue exposure.

Cue exposure, then, could be more usefully seen as a procedure for examining the nature of addiction. Drug cue exposure can result in autonomic, symbolic–expressive, and behavioural reactivity (Niaura et al., 1988; Drummond, Cooper & Glautier, 1990; Childress et al., 1988). Autonomic reactivity has been observed in cue exposure experiments with a wide range of drugs and has included effects on heart rate, pulse transit time, temperature, skin conductance, and salivation. Symbolic–expressive (or cognitive) reactivity has been found in terms of reported craving or urges to take drugs, in drug-related expectancies and self-efficacy beliefs, and more recently in information processing measures. Researchers have, on the basis of conditioning and cognitive theories, tended to make inferences about the likely behavioural consequences of these responses in terms of drug use. As more data have become available, however, the justification for these inferences has been called into question (see Glautier & Remington, Chapter 2; Tiffany, Chapter 3). Of the three types of cue reactivity, behavioural reactivity, or actual drug use following cue exposure, is the least studied, but is also the area which could potentially provide the most compelling evidence for the importance of cues in addiction.

The range of cues that may be relevant in addictive behaviours is potentially infinite. They include cues that occur before ingestion of a drug (exteroceptive cues), such as the sight, smell, and taste of a favourite alcoholic drink or cigarette, or the sight of a needle and syringe. More complex exteroceptive cues can involve the performance of a "cook-up" ritual, billboard alcohol advertising, or temporal cues such as the time of day when the drug is typically taken. Interoceptive cues can range from the sensation of a drug entering the stomach to the effects of a drug on neuroreceptors. Indeed, one dose of a drug may act as a cue for further drug ingestion, the so-called "priming dose effect" (or appetizer effect), which has been demonstrated in both alcohol-dependent and non-dependent subjects. Interoceptive cues can also include moods (such as euphoria or anger) and cognitions (such as beliefs about the effects of a drug). Finally, drug cues can be related to the withdrawal phase of the drug use cycle that can occur many hours after initial drug ingestion.

Individuals who exhibit addictive behaviour have had particular and extensive exposure to a wide range of cues associated with drug self-administration when compared to drug-naïve counterparts. General conditioning and cognitive theories provide specific predictions about the responses that an individual will exhibit both during and following drug cue exposure on the basis of that individual's past experience of the drug–cue pairings. This leads to the related question of what aspects of drug effect do cues become associated with? All drugs, by definition, have a pharmacological effect and therefore may promote conditioning. Psychoactive drugs, and in particular addictive drugs, have several properties with a high potential for conditioning (see Cami et al., 1991, for a review). First, all addictive drugs appear to operate as primary positive reinforcers: that is, animals will readily learn to self-administer these drugs. It is generally the case that stimuli that serve as reinforcers in instrumental conditioning support robust classical conditioning. Addictive drugs can also produce intensively positive hedonic mood effects, and many lead to dependence. The importance of dependence in this context lies in the regular occurrence of withdrawal effects that can be exhibited by intense negative affect and powerful physiological reactions. These strong physiological and psychological effects, and the ability of the drug to relieve them, are also good candidates for conditioning involvement.

The third use of the term "cue exposure" is in the context of a treatment approach to reduce or extinguish drug use. Again, conditioning theory has had an important influence in the development of this approach. When an animal is repeatedly exposed to a cue in the absence of drug ingestion, extinction of the CRs can take place. The cue no longer conveys the same information as it did during the acquisition phase of conditioning and so does not support further conditioned responding. This has led to the prediction that, in the drug-addicted individual, repeated, unreinforced exposure to drug cues should lead to extinction of CRs, which may reduce the likelihood of further drug self-administration. This has given rise to a wide range of investigations into cue exposure as a therapeutic technique in addictive behaviours (Childress et al., 1988; Drummond, Cooper & Glautier, 1990). Once again, while conditioning theory has been an important impetus in this area of cue exposure research, it is not necessarily the sole explanation for the effects of cue exposure treatment.

Most importantly, the cue exposure paradigm provides a crucial opportunity to make a connection between established general theories of behaviour and the understanding and treatment of the serious and growing public health problem of addiction. Unfortunately, the same could not be said for many of the therapeutic techniques commonly practised in the addictions field. It is in this way that cue exposure holds its greatest promise.

TO WHAT EXTENT IS CUE EXPOSURE A "NEW" APPROACH?

Cue exposure in relation to drugs has existed almost as long as classical conditioning theory itself. Krylov (in Pavlov, 1927) was the first to describe the acquisition of CRs to morphine cues in animals. This model was further developed by Wikler (1948) who proposed that drug cues had an important role in the basis of morphine addiction in both animals and humans. So the application of conditioning theories to drug taking has a long history. However, it was not until many years later that Wikler (1965) began to study cue exposure in relation to its therapeutic potential in addictive behaviours, and nearly 20 years after that when cue exposure was studied in a controlled trial with alcohol-dependent subjects (Rankin, Hodgson & Stockwell, 1983).

For several centuries the predominant approach to treatment of addictive behaviours has been that the addict should not only abstain from drugs but should avoid any exposure to the cues associated with drug use. Rush (1789) refers to the need for abstinence from alcohol and cue avoidance.

> It has been said, that the disuse of spirits should be gradual; but my observations authorise me to say, that persons who have been addicted to them, should abstain from them *suddenly* and *entirely.* "Taste not, handle not, touch not", should be enscribed on every vessel that contains spirits in the house of a man, who wishes to be cured of the habits of intemperance. (p. 341)

Interestingly, Rush's rationale for cue avoidance bears a remarkable similarity to modern concepts of cue reactivity.

> . . . that operation of the human mind, which obliges it to associate ideas, accidentally or otherwise combined, for the cure of vice, is very ancient. Our knowledge of this principle of association upon the minds and conduct of men, should lead us to destroy . . . the influence of all those circumstances, with which the recollection and desire of spirits are combined . . . and by restraining them . . . from those places and companions, which suggested to them the idea of ardent spirits, their habits of intemperance may be completely destroyed. (p. 340)

Cue avoidance has been particularly advocated in the treatment of alcohol dependence, and, to a large extent, remains a key element of alcoholism treatment programmes today. The Alcoholics Anonymous movement espouses this view particularly strongly, and most forms of residential treatment for alcoholism involve complete isolation from alcohol cues. So to suggest that, instead of avoiding cues, the addict should actually confront the cues associated with drug use, will be seen by many as a major departure from orthodoxy.

Conditioning theory-based treatments did enjoy a period of popularity in the addictions field in the 1970s in the form of aversive conditioning, often in the context of "controlled drinking" treatments. This involved the pairing of an addictive drug, typically alcohol, with an aversive stimulus such as an electric shock, aversive chemical agents, respiratory paralysis, or covert sensitization employing verbal aversion techniques (see Litman, 1976, for a review). Indeed, aversion therapy became a key element of many treatment programmes during the 1970s in the face of conflicting evidence of its effectiveness from controlled trials (Miller & Hester, 1986). Although there is now some evidence to suggest the utility of covert sensitization, aversion therapy has subsequently fallen into disuse partly through the controversy that surrounds the administration of alcohol to alcoholics, but perhaps mainly through the lack of acceptability of the technique to patients and therapists. It is important to note that cue exposure is not a reincarnation of aversive conditioning. While cue exposure may also to some extent be explained by conditioning theory it differs in respect of the method by which cues may be modified.

Cue exposure has already become established as the mainstay of treatment in phobic (Marks, 1987) and obsessional disorders (Rachman & Hodgson, 1980). Several controlled studies have demonstrated the effectiveness of this approach. Within this paradigm, the subject is exposed to the feared stimulus, such as a cat in the case of cat phobia (Freeman & Kendrick, 1960), as opposed to a drug cue in the drug-dependent individual, and the target response for extinction is an avoidant escape response rather than drug-taking behaviour. In a similar way obsessional neurosis has been treated successfully by exposure to the object of obsessions, such as dirt, whilst preventing a compulsive hand washing ritual from taking place. However, although there are many similarities between addictions and phobic and obsessional disorders it may be misleading to extrapolate the findings in the latter too far with regard to treatment efficacy. Nevertheless, the addictions field has much to learn from parallel studies in neurotic disorders.

So in conclusion, cue exposure is certainly not a new approach in understanding addictive behaviour, nor is it a new therapeutic technique. What is comparatively new is the systematic application of cue exposure as a treatment of addictions.

DO WE REALLY NEED ANOTHER MEANS OF UNDERSTANDING AND TREATING ADDICTION?

Cue exposure research must address two key questions. First, could it add anything to our current understanding of addiction, and second, do we need yet another treatment approach? In his 1988 editorial on the effectiveness of treatments for drinking problems Edwards states,

> If no treatment exists for a common and distressing condition that runs a fluctuating course, claims will abound for sovereign remedies. This has often been the case with inebriety [alcoholism] . . . As to what treatment

works for a high degree of [alcohol] dependence, here the debate is particularly open. (pp. 4–5)

The same view could be applied to the treatment of other common
addictive behaviours such as smoking and illicit drug use.

Further, Holder et al. (1991) in their study of cost effectiveness of alcoholism treatments noted that the predominant treatment modalities in the
US lacked evidence for their effectiveness and were amongst the most
costly. So there is not only a lack of consensus about the most effective
methods of treating alcoholism, but what research exists tends to be
ignored in practice. This situation can be seen in part as arising from the
absence of a leading theory of addiction and the difficulty in testing the
key elements of existing treatments.

This is the area in which cue exposure offers its greatest potential. In cue
exposure we have a means of developing an understanding of addictive
behaviour that is firmly rooted in widely studied general theories of
behaviour, theories that have been successfully applied to other areas of
human behavioural disorder. This in turn offers common ground for the
development of further research. Cue exposure provides a methodology
to test hypotheses of addictive behaviour through the application of
adequately controlled procedures. At a basic science level, we are able
to study mechanisms of drug tolerance, cue reactivity, and the effects of
cues on drug-seeking behaviour. These findings can then be applied to
those who suffer from addictions. In the clinical arena, cue exposure
allows a more precise method to study the phenomenon of relapse and,
ultimately, to study the effects of cue exposure on clinical outcome.

This is not to suggest that cue exposure should or even could corner the
market as a means of understanding or treating addictions. Just as there
is danger in ignorance and confusion, so there is equal danger in the
simple-minded application of scientific theories. Rather, cue exposure
should be seen as providing another means of studying addictive behaviour, of generating new hypotheses which can be tested, and producing
findings which can be debated, replicated, or refuted. Addiction is a complex bio-psycho-social phenomenon which defies simple accounts or sol-
utions.

The cue exposure paradigm should not be seen as being in competition
with leading theories of addiction. Cue reactivity research can, however,
be used to extend research in a wide range of theoretical models. The
aim here is not to provide an exhaustive list of models to which the cue
exposure paradigm can be applied, but rather to provide examples to
illustrate key issues. Genetic research has become an important

developing area in recent years, although evidence for the role of genetic factors in the addictions has, so far, been limited (Peters & Edwards, 1994). Part of the problem may lie in the looseness of the definitions of what it is that is inherited. The phenotype is typically defined as "alcoholism" or "drug addiction", which, are themselves, highly complex phenomena. The introduction of standard definitions used specifically in the addictions field to describe the target behaviours may help this line of research. A potential application of cue exposure in this area is in studying the effects of exposure to drug-related cues between different generations, and in studying the responses to drug cues in children of drug-dependent and non-drug-dependent parents. Differences between children of alcoholic and non-alcoholic parents have been found in subjective effects of ethanol (Schuckit, 1984), in electroencephalography (Gabrielli et al., 1982), evoked potentials (Begleiter et al., 1984), body sway (Schuckit, 1985), and certain biological markers (Schuckit, Gold & Risch, 1987). Importantly for cue exposure, differences in responsivity of non-alcoholic sons of alcoholic and non-alcohlic fathers have been found. For example, Newlin (1985) found that sons of alcoholic fathers had enhanced "antagonistic placebo responses" to alcohol cues, similar to those found in heavy drinkers. Such research suggests that cue exposure investigations may provide specific and more accurately measurable phenomena that may be relevant to the heritability of addictive behaviour (see Rees & Heather, Chapter 5).

Although the disease concept of alcoholism in reality represents a conglomeration of different theoretical and clinical concepts gathered over the years, and is therefore difficult to test or falsify, it is possible to examine certain aspects of disease theory from the perspective of the cue exposure paradigm. One key feature which may at first appear incompatible with cue exposure when applied as a therapeutic procedure, is the importance of cue avoidance as advocated by AA or Narcotics Anonymous. However, it is perhaps not surprising that an abstinent addict exposed to drug cues in the naturalistic setting may be overwhelmed by their responses and relapse to drug taking. This underscores the potential importance of cue reactivity in relapse and the need to expose a subject to cues gradually and, initially at least, in a more controlled and supportive environment. Cue reactivity also provides a possible explanation for the tenets, "one drink, one drunk", and "once an alcoholic, always an alcoholic", particularly where the treatment programme does not prepare individuals for their almost inevitable encounter with alcohol-related cues after leaving a residential treatment setting.

Social learning theory has recently provided rich new directions in understanding and treating addictive behaviours. Here too, cue exposure offers a means to extend research in this area. Marlatt (1985) proposed that when an abstinent alcoholic encounters a "high risk situation", in effect, one which involves exposure to salient drug use cues, there will be an increased likelihood of relapse compared with other situations. The alcoholic's "outcome expectancies" (beliefs concerning the consequences of taking alcohol) and "self-efficacy" (the extent to which they believe they can resist the temptation to drink alcohol) will determine whether relapse occurs in this situation. The cue exposure paradigm allows another means to test this theory. With cue exposure it is possible to recreate, to a large extent, the setting in which an individual has in the past relapsed, and to study the processes that might be responsible.

In summary, we do need the development of new theories and new theory-based treatments in the addictions, particularly in an area that is short of hypotheses that can be tested and treatments that can be adequately evaluated. However, instead of putting forward one theoretical framework to the exclusion of all others, we propose that cue exposure is a valuable investigative technique that can be studied from a variety of different theoretical standpoints. General theories of behaviour are likely to be more useful candidates for such investigation than those which are substance or behaviour specific. This is more in keeping with a broader movement towards finding commonalities between addictions rather than differences (Marks, 1990).

WHERE ARE WE IN THE DEVELOPMENT OF CUE EXPOSURE RESEARCH AND PRACTICE?

Although the cue exposure paradigm has been in existence for many years, it is only relatively recently that it has begun to gather momentum in addictions research. In such a developing field it is important not to overstate the position and to rush prematurely into advocating a major departure from usual practice. This is particularly true in the field of addiction treatment where history cautions against overstatement. Such action would only be a disservice to the progress that has been achieved since Wikler drew attention to drug cue reactivity phenomena. We aim here to provide a broad overview of the status of the cue exposure field. In stepping back from the detail, we will identify areas of progress as well as important areas that are, so far, relatively unexplored.

Over the last decade there has been a rapid increase in the information available on cue reactivity from both animal and human laboratories and in the clinical research field. The topics covered in this book are divided into three main areas:

1. Theoretical issues in drug cue exposure;
2. Methods of studying human drug cue reactivity;
3. Clinical applications of cue exposure in addictive behaviour.

We will now look at each area in turn.

Theoretical Issues in Drug Cue Exposure

A great deal of research in this field has focused on studying the extent to which responses to drug cues provide evidence to support conditioning accounts of addictive behaviour. Considerable research has investigated the direction of responses to cues. Responses have been proposed to be either withdrawal-like (Wikler, 1948), drug-like (Stewart, de Wit & Eikelboom, 1984), or drug-opposite (Siegel, 1975). After reviewing this research, Glautier & Remington (Chapter 2) conclude that, while such monistic models of the form of response to drug cues have been influential in the development of the drug cue exposure research field, the available data do not support one model to the exclusion of all others. Moreover, it is not possible to draw inferences about the behavioural effects of cue exposure on the basis of the psychological or physiological state of the organism in any reliable way. Instead, they propose that the key variable of interest in studying cue reactivity should be drug-seeking behaviour since this is of greatest relevance to addictive behaviour as it is the final common pathway through which cue reactivity is channelled.

Similarly, Tiffany (Chapter 3) proposes that theories of interaction between classical and operant conditioning, which have been influential in the development of drug cue exposure research, have been superseded by developments in the broader field of conditioning research. Much debate in the cue exposure field has centred around whether drug taking is motivated by positive or negative reinforcement, whereas in reality, the situation is likely to be much more complex. Not only is relief of conditioned withdrawal, for example, likely to be too simple as a model of the way in which cues motivate drug use, but the idea that discrete CRs lead to changes in operant behaviour has been hard to sustain. Two-process theories of the interaction between operant and classical conditioning were replaced by the concept of central emotional states as mediators of instrumental behaviour over 20 years ago (Rescorla & Solomon, 1967).

So, is it the case that studies into the nature of cue reactivity conducted thus far have been a wasted effort? Certainly results would suggest that attempts to explain fully drug cue reactivity phenomena in terms of conditioning theory have not so far been successful. Any further research in this area must take account of advances in general conditioning and cognitive theories of behaviour, a link which has not always been made successfully. However, the utility of cue exposure does not rely on support from basic conditioning research. Instead it is up to conditioning research to prove its utility in explaining cue reactivity phenomena. Importantly, the most critical research in studying the potential link between cue reactivity and drug-taking behaviour has yet to be conducted. Further, it is not the case that there is a complete absence of data to support a conditioning account of cue reactivity. Rather, there is evidence to suggest that it is relevant to drug taking behaviour, but simple models have proved to be inadequate.

Methods of Studying Human Drug Cue Reactivity

Here too, there is some convergence towards a consensus of the current status of cue reactivity research. Much of the cue reactivity research so far conducted in this field has relied on subjects' assumed extra-experimental experience with drugs. Thus, most of this research has drawn inferences from comparisons between drug-dependent and non-dependent individuals, or in differences in reactivity to neutral and drug-related cues in dependent individuals. Again, there is conflicting evidence concerning the validity of both conditioning and cognitive accounts of the underlying processes. This is in part due to the fact that many studies have not employed adequate control procedures for assessing cue reactivity. Glautier & Tiffany (Chapter 4) and Greeley & Ryan (Chapter 6) both refer to the importance of applying Robbins & Ehrman's (1992) criteria in assessing and designing human drug-conditioning experiments, criteria that relate mainly to selection of controls. Further, there is a call for standardization and improvement in measurement, particularly the assessment of craving, which, until recently, has tended to be carried out with single-item measures.

Glautier & Tiffany (Chapter 4) argue that a key methodological advance in cue exposure research is in studies which control for extra-experimental experience with drug cues, where individuals are conditioned to novel drug cues in a controlled environment. An example of this is Glautier, Drummond & Remington's (1994) study in which non-dependent drinkers acquired CRs to novel stimuli signalling alcohol delivery. In this way it is possible to isolate the effects of conditioning from the myriad of influences on reactivity in clinical populations of addicts. However, the utility of this approach in explaining addictive behaviour in addict populations, and in demonstrating the effect of conditioned cues on drug-seeking behaviour, remains some way off.

Another example of increasing sophistication in theory and research methods comes from Tiffany's (Chapter 7) account of the development of cognitive models to study cue reactivity. Once again, it appears that simplistic models of craving *causing* relapse are inadequate to explain the phenomena. Instead, Tiffany cites his cognitive processing model of cue reactivity (Tiffany, 1990) which distinguishes between automatic and non-automatic processes in the regulation of drug-taking behaviour. In this model, reactivity to cues reflects, in large part, the immediate cognitive and behavioural demands of the situation, and is not a direct manifestation of classically conditioned responses. Although this model has many advantages in explaining some of the discrepant findings in cue reactivity research, it requires further support from empirical research. Most importantly, however, it opens a new area of research enquiry into cue reactivity.

The use of group designs to study cue reactivity has been the mainstay of previous research, but the study of individual differences (Rees & Heather, Chapter 5) holds promise in developing models of cue reactivity and clinical methods to assess and treat addictive behaviour. The fact that certain individuals react more strongly to cues than others opens a range of questions concerning individual susceptibility to addiction. Rees & Heather cite several examples where cue reactivity research may have an important role in genetic and personality research in the addiction field. Again, the value of cue reactivity research in this context does not require conditioning theory to account for the findings, although individual differences in conditionability to cues provides a rich area of testable hypotheses. Of greater practical importance is the study of individual differences in cue reactivity in assessment and treatment of addictive behaviour, an issue that is discussed in the next section. If certain individuals are more susceptible to relapse by virtue of greater cue reactivity, then the measurement of cue reactivity may have practical utility in screening for those at higher risk of relapse and, ultimately, in preventing relapse.

Clinical Applications of Cue Exposure in Addictive Behaviour

Many advances have been made recently in clinical research in the cue exposure field, but the message from this area must be that we still have some way to go in providing effective, practical methods to treat addictive behaviours. There have now been several demonstrations of a connection between cue reactivity and relapse to both smoking and alcohol use following a period of abstinence that adds support to the view of Ludwig, Wikler & Stark (1974) that,

> ... any therapeutic approach ... that does not recognise the powerful, evocative effects of interoceptive and exteroceptive stimuli ... and that neglects to provide techniques for modifying the strength of these effects will likely be destined to failure. (p. 547)

While we do not completely endorse this view, there is now a growing body of research suggesting that, in spite of technical difficulties is explaining cue reactivity solely in terms of conditioning or cognitive theories, cue reactivity is a clinically relevant phenomenon.

There are also now a number of demonstrations that cue exposure treatment can modify relapse in addictive behaviour (Rohsenow, Monti & Abrams, Chapter 8). The evidence is stronger in the area of alcohol dependence than in opiate and cocaine (Dawe & Powell, Chapter 9) or nicotine dependence (Brandon et al., Chapter 10). This is, in part, related to the greater amount of clinical research in cue exposure that has so far been conducted in the alcohol dependence field. The positive findings from alcohol research should provide a stimulus for further research with other substances.

There is a great deal to be learned from other areas of research in further developing cue exposure as a clinical technique in addictive behaviour. Several authors point to the advances made in the treatment of phobic and obsessional behaviours while cautioning against making too great a leap of faith in assuming their equivalence to addictive behaviours. We need to move forward from conducting cue exposure in the laboratory setting towards employing cues that are as close to the real life drug-taking situation as possible. In selected groups, this may include providing access to the drug itself as has been done in the smoking field (Brandon et al., Chapter 10). Any procedure of this sort, however, must take account of the risk of relapse during treatment if the individual is inadequately supported or if the cues are overwhelming in salience and intensity. Gradually increasing intensity of exposure is more likely to be successful than flooding in this context.

We need to get better at selecting individuals who are more likely to benefit from cue exposure, and each of the treatment chapters provides useful pointers in this respect. As suggested earlier, identifying individuals who are more reactive to cues is likely to be one important approach. It will also be important to tailor cue exposure more to individual needs than has been the case so far, a point that can be learned from the phobic and obsessional cue exposure fields. From the addicted individual's perspective, we must develop treatment techniques that are perceived as being relevant to his or her problem, rather than relying on methods suggested by theory. Further, as anxiety and affective disorders often co-exist with addictions, we should be looking towards cue exposure treatments that more effectively address the problems of co-morbidity.

Another clinical reality that must be addressed by the cue exposure field is the issue of cost effectiveness (Holder et al., 1991). In an era when cost containment is a key priority in health-care delivery, we must look to developing methods that are practicable in the real world. If cue exposure treatment can be delivered only by highly trained clinicians in well-equipped clinical facilities, then cue exposure treatment may find only limited application in spite of positive results. However, it is important to remember that cue exposure is at a very early stage of development as a clinical procedure. We might learn from the area of cue exposure for phobic and obsessional behaviours that it may take several years for treatment methods to become more widely applicable and delivered by less specialized professionals than is the case during development. The main priority of the field at present is to establish whether cue exposure can be effective and to define the optimal methods of delivery. Brandon and colleagues (Chapter 10) also draw attention to the importance of the "stepped care approach" (Lichtenstein & Hollis, 1992; Orleans, 1993) in the smoking field where progression to more intensive interventions is determined by response to more minimal interventions: it would be inappropriate to advocate intensive cue exposure as a first treatment option in every case.

MAKING THE CONNECTION BETWEEN BASIC AND CLINICAL CUE EXPOSURE RESEARCH

Looking at the evidence from basic and clinical drug cue exposure research in the round we conclude that the greatest challenge at present is to make the connection between advances in all areas rather than the somewhat focused approach that has existed thus far. Basic research on drug cue exposure has to examine questions that address the clinical realities of the addicted individual. Similarly, clinical research on cue exposure must take greater account of advances in basic cue reactivity research. While the clinical application of cue exposure does not stand or fall on the success or failure of basic animal or human experiments to explain cue reactivity phenomena in terms of conditioning, cognitive, or indeed other general theories of behaviour, clinical research has much to learn from basic research.

Much of the clinical cue exposure research conducted thus far has been driven by theoretical models of cue reactivity that are outdated and no longer applicable. However, rather than detracting from the clinical advances that have been made, new knowledge of the nature and mechanism of cue reactivity provides important new directions for clinical research. The increasing interest in and relevance of clinical cue exposure research, in spite of conflicting and sometimes discouraging basic research, is testament to the perceived clinical relevance of cue reactivity, regardless of how it may be explained. However, as pointed out recently there is a danger in moving forward too quickly with clinical trials of cue exposure in advance of necessary developmental work on mechanisms of cue reactivity (Drummond et al., 1990). Negative findings may serve only to inappropriately divert attention from what is a promising line of enquiry. As Brandon et al. (Chapter 10) suggest, we need to refine our methods before moving towards large-scale clinical trials.

Nevertheless, methods can be refined in the context of clinical trials. Clinical research in cue exposure needs to incorporate greater enquiry into the mechanism and process of treatment as much as studying outcome. Recent studies have demonstrated the way in which cue reactivity can be used to examine the process of treatment in the context of clinical trials (Drummond & Glautier, 1994; Monti et al., 1993). With increasing sophistication in our understanding and measurement of cue reactivity, we have an opportunity to develop clinical techniques that are both rich in information about the processes and mechanisms involved, and are, at the same time, grounded in science.

The principal aim of this book is to open greater dialogue between basic and clinical scientists in the drug cue exposure field. Clinical and basic research cannot and should not occur in separate vacua. Each field needs to take more account of the other. The detailed reviews of each area together aim to provide an overall view of the current state of the art. A further aim has been to stimulate interest in cue exposure as method to study and treat addictive behaviours. We hope the advances described here will stimulate cue exposure research to investigate the directions suggested here. We also suggest that the drug cue exposure paradigm will be recognized as an increasingly attractive method to study basic principles of human behaviour. Not only does cue exposure provide a means to study and treat addictive behaviours, drug cue exposure provides a means to study behaviour itself.

At the same time we caution against research that is out of step with the clinical realities of addictive behaviour. Addictions provide an enormous source of morbidity and distress in society. Cue exposure should not be seen as being a panacea in terms of either explanation or solution. Rather, we present cue exposure as a promising means of continuing the long march of progress in the development of scientifically-based approaches to understanding and treating addictions.

REFERENCES

Begleiter, H., Porjesz, B., Bihari, B. & Kissin, B. (1984). Event-related brain potentials in boys at risk for alcoholism. *Science*, **225**, 1493–1496.

Cami, J., Bigelow, G.E., Griffiths, R.R. & Drummond, D.C. (1991). Clinical testing of drug abuse liability. *British Journal of Addiction*, **86**, 1525–1652.

Childress, A.R., McLellan, A.T., Ehrman, R. & O'Brien, C.P. (1988). Classically conditioned responses in opioid and cocaine dependence: a role in relapse? In *Learning Factors in Substance Abuse, NIDA Research Monograph 84*, pp. 25–43. Washington, DC: Department of Health and Human Services.

Drummond, D.C. & Glautier, S. (1994). A controlled trial of cue exposure treatment in alcohol dependence. *Journal of Consulting and Clinical Psychology*, **62**, 809–817.

Drummond, D.C., Cooper, T. & Glautier, S.P. (1990). Conditioned learning in alcohol dependence: implications for cue exposure treatment. *British Journal of Addiction*, **85**, 725–743.

Edwards, G. (1988) What treatments work for drinking problems? *British Medical Journal*, **296**, 4–5.

Freeman, H.L. & Kendrick, D.C. (1960). A case of cat phobia. *British Medical Journal*, **ii**, 497–502.

Gabrielli, W.F., Mednick, S.A., Volvaka, J., Pollock, V.E., Schulsinger, F. & Itil, T.M. (1982). Electroencephalograms in children of alcoholic fathers. *Psychophysiology*, **19**, 404–407.

Glautier, S., Drummond, D.C. & Remington, B. (1994). Alcohol as an unconditioned stimulus in human classical conditioning. *Psychopharamacology*, **116**, 360–368.

Holder, H., Longabaugh, R., Miller, W.R. & Rubonis, A.V. (1991). The cost effectiveness of treatment for alcoholism: a first approximation. *Journal of Studies on Alcohol*, **52**, 517–539.

Lichtenstein, E. & Hollis, J. (1992). Patient referral to a smoking cessation program: who follows through? *Journal of Family Practice*, **34**, 739–744.

Litman, G.K. (1976). Behavioural modification techniques in the treatment of alcoholism: a review and critique. In Gibbins et al. (Eds), *Alcohol*, Vol. 3. New York: Wiley.

Ludwig, A.M., Wikler, A. & Stark, L.H. (1974). The first drink: psychobiological aspects of craving. *Archives of General Psychiatry*, **30**, 539–547.

Marlatt, G.A. (1985). Situational determinants of relapse and skill-training interventions. In Marlatt, G.A. & Gordon, J.R. (Eds), *Relapse Prevention: Maintenance Strategies in the Treatment of Addictive Behaviors*. New York: Guilford.

Marks, I.M. (1987). *Fears, Phobias and Rituals*. New York: Oxford University Press.

Marks, I.M. (1990). Behavioural (non-chemical) addictions. *British Journal of Addiction*, **85**, 1389–1394.

Miller, W.R. & Hester, R.K. (1986). The effectiveness of alcoholism treatment: what research reveals. In Miller, W.R. & Heather, N. (Eds), *Treating Addictive Behaviours: Processes of Change*. New York: Plenum.

Monti, P.M., Rohsenow, D.J., Rubonis, A.V., Niaura, R.S., Sirota, A.D., Colby, S.M., Goddard, P. & Abrams, D.B. (1993). Cue exposure with coping skills treatment for male alcoholics: a preliminary investigation. *Journal of Consulting and Clinical Psychology*, **61**, 1011–1019.

Newlin, D.B. (1985). Offspring of alcoholics have enhanced antagonistic placebo response. *Journal of Studies on Alcohol*, **46**, 490–494.

Niaura, R.S., Rosenhow, D.J., Binkoff, J.A., Monti, P.M., Pedraza, M. & Abrams, D.B. (1988). Relevance of cue reactivity to understanding alcohol and smoking relapse. *Journal of Abnormal Psychology*, **97**, 133–152.

Orleans, T.C. (1993). Treating nicotine dependence in medical settings: a stepped-care model. In Orleans, C.T. & Slade, J. (Eds), *Nicotine Addiction: Principles and Management*. Cambridge: Cambridge University Press.

Pavlov, I.P. (1927). *Conditioned Reflexes* (reprinted 1960). New York: Dover Publications.

Peters, T.J. & Edwards, G. (1994). Introduction: finding new directions. In Peters, T.J. & Edwards, G. (Eds), Alcohol and alcohol problems. *British Medical Bulletin*, **50**, 1–4.

Rachman, S. & Hodgson, R. (1980). *Obsessions and Compulsions*. Englewood-Cliffs, NJ: Prentice Hall.

Rankin, H., Hodgson, R. & Stockwell, T. (1983). Cue exposure and response prevention with alcoholics: a controlled trial. *Behaviour Research and Therapy*, **21**, 435–446.

Rescorla, R.A. & Solomon, R.L. (1967). Two-process learning theory: relationships between Pavlovian conditioning and instrumental learning. *Psychological Review*, **74**, 151–182.

Robbins, S.J. & Ehrman, R.N. (1992). Designing studies of drug conditioning in humans. *Psychopharmacology*, **106**, 143–153.

Rush, B. (1789) *An Inquiry Into the Effects of Ardent Spirits Upon the Human Body and Mind with an Account of the Means of Preventing Them and of the Remedies for Curing Them*, 8th edn (reprinted 1814). Brookfield: Merriam.

Schuckit, M.A. (1984). Subjective responses to alcohol in sons of alcoholics and control subjects. *Archives of General Psychiatry*, **41**, 879–884.

Schuckit, M.A. (1985). Ethanol-induced changes in body sway in men at high alcoholism risk. *Archives of General Psychiatry*, **42**, 375–379.

Schuckit, M.A., Gold, E. & Risch, C. (1987). Serum prolactin levels in sons of alcoholics and control subjects. *American Journal of Psychiatry*, **144**, 854–859.

Siegel, S. (1975). Evidence from rats that morphine tolerance is a learned response. *Journal of Comparative and Physiological Psychology*, **89**, 498–506.

Stewart, J., de Wit, H. & Eikelboom, R. (1984). Role of unconditioned and conditioned drug effects in the self administration of opiates and stimulants. *Psychological Review*, **91**, 251–268.

Tiffany, S.T. (1990). A cognitive model of drug urges and drug-use behaviour: the role of automatic and non-automatic processes. *Psychological Review*, **97**, 147–168.

Wikler, A. (1948). Recent progress in research on the neurophysiologic basis of morphine addiction. *American Journal of Psychiatry*, **105**, 329–338.

Wikler, A. (1965). Conditioning factors in opiate addiction and relapse. In Wiher, D.I. & Kassebaum, G. (Eds), *Narcotics*. New York: McGraw-Hill.

SECTION I

The Theoretical Basis of Cue Exposure in Addictive Behaviour

CHAPTER 2   The form of responses to drug cues

Steven Glautier and
Bob Remington†*

INTRODUCTION

Human drug-seeking behaviour is a prototypical example of operant behaviour; much human and animal behaviour is operant, in the sense that it can be interpreted as a function of its environmental consequences. The consequence of a particular act may increase or sustain the subsequent likelihood of the act, in which case the consequence is called a reinforcer, or reduce its subsequent likelihood, in which case it is called a punisher. The behaviours leading up to drug consumption are operant in the sense that they are under the control of the reinforcing consequences of drug self-administration. In general, self-administered drugs are said to have positive hedonic effects (positive reinforcement) and/or to relieve or prevent aversive states (negative reinforcement). Although some authors have stressed the importance of positive reinforcement in the maintenance of drug use (e.g. Stewart, de Wit & Eikelboom, 1984; Wise & Bozarth, 1987), whereas others have stressed the role of negative reinforcement (e.g. Edwards, 1990), both of these processes probably play a part in the maintenance of drug use.

Given the strength of an operant interpretation of drug-seeking behaviour, one may legitimately wonder what relevance classical, or Pavlovian, conditioning has in this context. In a typical classical conditioning experiment, a subject is presented with a stimulus, such as a light, and shortly afterwards a second more potent stimulus follows (for example, a startlingly loud noise). After a number of such co-presentations, the subject's behaviour with respect to the light changes markedly. The objective of such an experiment is to study how the relationship between

---

*National Addiction Centre, University of London, UK and †University of Southampton, UK

Addictive Behaviour: Cue Exposure Theory and Practice.
Edited by D.C. Drummond, S.T. Tiffany, S. Glautier and B. Remington.
© 1995 John Wiley & Sons Ltd.

the first and second stimulus affects behaviour occurring during the first, "signal", stimulus. The behavioural changes seen may be physiological (e.g. a racing heart), behavioural (e.g. cringing away from the light), or cognitive (e.g. thinking that the light is bad, or sinister). Rescorla has provided a definition of classical conditioning in the following terms:

> Classical conditioning is said to have occurred if a measurable change in an organism's behaviour to a conditioned stimulus (CS) can be attributed to the relationship between that stimulus and an unconditioned stimulus (US). (Rescorla, 1988, p. 152)

The response to the CS is called the conditioned response (CR) while the response to the US is known as an unconditioned response (UR).

Why should classical conditioning be relevant to the operant behaviours involved in drug self-administration? The answer to this question lies in the following facts. First, in any operant learning situation, there is a strong possibility that classical conditioning may occur adventitiously, and second, the conditioned responses which develop may in some way moderate the occurrence of the operant behaviour. For example, suppose a heroin user regularly self-administers a dose of the drug in a particular location, close to where the drug is obtained. Seeking out and injecting the drug is clearly operant, maintained by the reinforcing effects of the injection, but the act of injection necessarily means that the user experiences drug effects in the presence of distinctive cues arising from the location, the needle and syringe, and so on. Because a drug such as heroin has powerful discriminative and hedonic effects, it has the capacity to act as a US and thus, cues which are regularly associated with this US can acquire CS functions. It might be expected, therefore, that drug users' purposive operant behaviour, in particular their drug seeking and administration, would be affected should they experience these cues again at some point in the future.

Notice that, like Rescorla's definition of classical conditioning, this example is silent about the precise nature of the changes in behaviour brought about through the association of events described. One aim of this chapter is to describe the kinds of behavioural change that have been observed when drug-based CSs are presented, and to see how well the data relate to existing theoretical accounts of the form of the CR in drug conditioning. We will show that none of the major models of response form can be excluded, nor are any adequate to account for all data. Another aim of the chapter is to present evidence that various features of USs and CSs need to be taken into account if predictions of CR form are to be made. For example, USs produce very complex kinds of behavioural change, and responses to signals for those USs reflect this fact.

However, none of the existing models of response form take these features into account and this may well account for their apparent shortcomings. Thus, with current knowledge in classical conditioning it is impossible to do more than to raise these features as issues to be considered in relation to the prediction of CR form. We will therefore not attempt to construct a detailed model of how the various factors may interact. Before embarking on the analysis, however, it is important to show that there is empirical evidence (a) for the fact that a drug can indeed act as a US in a classical conditioning study, and (b) that a drug-related CS can in practice alter the course of drug-seeking operant behaviour.

Drug-based Classical Conditioning

In a recent study lasting for several experimental sessions, healthy human volunteer subjects repeatedly consumed distinctively coloured and flavoured alcoholic and soft drinks (Glautier, Drummond & Remington, 1994). On any particular session subjects got either alcohol or soft drink and, since the psychological and physiological consequences of consuming the drinks differed, it was hypothesized that the colour and flavour of the alcoholic drink would acquire excitatory conditioned stimulus properties (CS+) in comparison to the soft drink (CS−). What was of special interest was the subjects' reactions to the presentation of a drink at the start of each session. Alcohol was always given in a red angostura mixture whereas soft drink was always presented as a blue peppermint soft mixture.[1] A key dependent variable was the skin conductance responses to the initial presentation of the drinks. It was found that habituation to the presentation of the soft drink occurred readily over sessions, but there was no corresponding habituation to the alcoholic drink. The responses to the visual presentation of these drinks over the course conditioning blocks are illustrated in Figure 2.1. The differential responsiveness to CS+ and CS− for alcohol can be attributed to the relationship between those cues and the drug's effect. In other words, the skin conductance responses observed meet Rescorla's definition of classical conditioning, and the study shows that drug-based conditioning does indeed occur in normal subjects with a commonly used legal drug.

CS-induced Modification of Drug-seeking Behaviour

It is substantially harder to show that classical CSs can modify the ongoing operant behaviour of human subjects. There is, however, good evi-

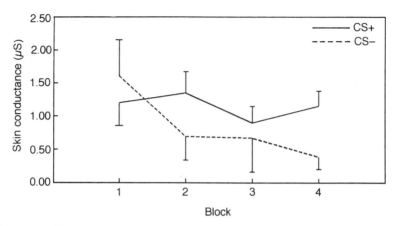

Figure 2.1 Skin conductance responses to the first sight of distinctive alcoholic (CS+) or soft (CS−) drinks over the course of conditioning blocks (1–4) as subjects gained experience of the relationship between drink colour and alcoholic contents. See text for a description of the experiment.

dence for such an effect from the animal laboratory. For example, Goldberg, Woods & Schuster (1969) trained morphine-dependent monkeys to press a lever to obtain a small dose of morphine. Clearly, this is a case of operant conditioning in that a response class, lever pressing, is under the control of its consequences, a dose of morphine. When nalorphine, a morphine antagonist, was given to these monkeys via injection it produced increases in lever pressing. In other words, nalorphine increased the reward value of the morphine as indexed by the fact that the animals worked harder to obtain the same dose. More important in this context, however, was the demonstration that increases in lever pressing could also be produced by presentation of a CS (illumination of a light) that had been paired with the nalorphine infusion. Since it is likely that the light acquired its effects because of its close association with the effects of the nalorphine injection, once again the change in function of the light meets Rescorla's defining conditions for classical conditioning and this study shows how a drug CS can moderate operant drug-seeking behaviour.

The demonstrable close connection between operant and classical conditioning leads quite naturally to a consideration of how the two processes interact with one another to bring about the smooth dynamics of behaviour we see in everyday life. Three basic accounts of the way that Pavlovian CSs can control drug-taking behaviour have been offered (i.e. Wikler, 1948; Siegel, 1975; Stewart, de Wit & Eikelboom, 1984). Although each proposes that the occurrence of stimuli with drug CS properties during drug-taking episodes will serve to increase the likelihood of drug use, they differ in terms of the manner in which these cues are supposed to function. At the heart of each model lies the assumption that the observed form of CRs elicited by drug cues can provide clues to the nature of their motivational function, and the form of these CRs is described by simple reference to the URs elicited by the drug. Thus, CRs are said either (a) to resemble an unconditioned drug withdrawal state (Wikler, 1948), (b) to resemble the unconditioned effects of the drug itself (Stewart, de Wit & Eikelboom, 1984), or (c) to oppose the unconditioned effects of the drug itself (Siegel, 1975). Typically, these CRs are changes in physiological response systems such as heart rate, skin conductance, skin temperature and so on, but other subjective and behavioural measures have also been used. Before questioning the adequacy of these rather simple formulations, we will provide a brief description of the three basic accounts, and of some of the data ostensibly providing support for each model.

ACCOUNTS OF DRUG CONDITIONING EFFECTS

There is now a large and extremely complex database relevant to assessing the veracity of the three basic models of CR form. We will make no attempt at a review; for more extensive analysis the reader is referred to Niaura et al. (1988), Siegel (1989), Drummond, Cooper & Glautier (1990) and Powell et al. (1990). Overall, our purpose is to argue that there are data to be found in support of each model, and that any model that predicts CRs to have one form or another is oversimplified. There are several reasons for this. First, as we indicate in the succeeding paragraphs, there may be considerable difficulties distinguishing between drug-like, drug-opposite, and drug-withdrawal responses to drug cues on physiological measures. In addition, as we will argue in the second half of the chapter, prediction US–UR is hindered by the complex nature of the US–UR relationship, and because the type of CS itself can influence the form of CR. In the brief review that follows we will consider two kinds of experiment, namely opportunistic experiments and conditioning experiments. An example of a conditioning experiment was given in the Introduction (Glautier, Drummond & Remington, 1994; their defining feature is that the experimenter actually arranges a conditioning procedure. In contrast, in an opportunistic experiment, the experimenter does not carry out conditioning but selects subjects who have an extra-experimental conditioning history. For example, heroin injectors and healthy controls may both be presented with needles and syringes and differences in their responses to these stimuli monitored.

However, generally speaking, opportunistic experiments are a weaker form of evidence since in many cases it is not clear what factors cause the putative drug CS to elicit responses which differ from those elicited by control stimuli (see Glautier and Tiffany, this volume, Chapter 4, for a detailed discussion of opportunistic and conditioning experiment design).

Models of Response Form

Wikler (1948) proposed that addiction to morphine was maintained by two sources of reinforcement; the direct pleasurable effects of the drug, and the satisfaction derived from morphine's ability to reduce distress arising from withdrawal and from other sources. However, he also sought to explain why relapse to drug use was so likely following abatement of acute withdrawal symptoms, i.e. when one of the main motivators of drug use had been removed. In answering this question, Wikler developed the conditioned withdrawal model, which has become the single most influential approach to the role of classical conditioning in the maintenance of drug use. Although some of the details and emphases have changed in his later formulations, the essential point has remained. Wikler believed that various kinds of cues for drug use elicited CRs resembling morphine withdrawal symptoms, and relapse after a period of abstinence could be motivated by the desire to relieve these conditioned withdrawal symptoms. In order to explain how withdrawal symptoms could be conditioned to cues for drug use, Wikler turned to traditional conditioning preparations for examples. In appetitive conditioning with a food US, which is perhaps a close parallel to the drug-taking situation, the immediate sensory events associated with the US being placed in the mouth are accompanied by adaptive responses, including salivation and stomach acid secretion. Wikler considered that the CRs elicited by a drug CS would resemble the later adaptive responses to the drug rather than the immediate sensory drug effects. By adaptive responses, Wikler meant the state of disequilibrium that occurs on drug withdrawal, particularly for physically dependent individuals. Therefore, he expected drug CSs to elicit CRs resembling withdrawal states rather than immediate drug effects.

In a model similar to Wikler's, Siegel (1975; see Siegel, 1989, for a recent and thorough review) proposed that the responses elicited by drug CSs will oppose the unconditioned immediate effects of the drug (in contrast to resembling later withdrawal effects). The model is generally known as the conditioned opponent process or conditioned compensatory response model and is related to more general opponent process accounts of learning (e.g. Solomon & Corbit, 1973, 1974; Schull, 1979; Wagner, 1981). The similarities to Wikler's model are especially apparent in two ways. First, when a drug has a biphasic action, i.e. when its initial and later effects are in opposite directions, then the predictions of the models are the same. Second, both models incorporate a drive reduction process since in both cases it is argued that negative reinforcement is the primary mechanism by which CRs to drug cues modulate drug taking. It is assumed that conditioned opponent processes are aversive, as are conditioned withdrawal symptoms, and this aversive state is reduced by drug taking. In fact, Poulos, Hinson & Siegel (1981) and Siegel (1989) have argued that "withdrawal symptoms" in general may be more properly termed drug-opposite preparatory responses. One essential feature of Siegel's model is the idea that the expression of tolerance to drug actions is affected by the presence of CSs for drug delivery, and it is argued that the drug-opposite CRs sum with the drug URs to produce this conditioned tolerance effect.

Next to the two drive reduction models just described we can juxtapose the model of drug-like CRs to drug CSs put forward by Stewart, de Wit & Eikelboom (1984). The well-known phrases "one drink, one drunk" or "one drink away from a drunk" reflect a widespread belief that when a dependent drinker consumes a small dose of alcohol, further and excessive drinking inevitably ensues. As described below, there is reasonable evidence for the fact that a small priming dose of a drug can directly increase the probability of further drug use. Since presentation of a drug cue may also have this effect, and based on evidence that similar neural mechanisms may underlie both effects, Stewart, de Wit & Eikelboom (1984) have proposed that the CRs elicited by drug CSs resemble, rather than oppose, drug effects or resemble drug withdrawal states. It is argued that drug CSs act as conditioned reinforcers or conditioned incentive stimuli, sharing the positive affective attributes of immediate drug effects.

Opportunistic Experiments

As mentioned above, the presentation of evidence in favour of the three models of response will be done under two headings. In this section opportunistic experiments will be described. This class of experiment is generally less satisfactory than conditioning experiments since there may be many reasons for suspecting that differences in the responses elicited by putative drug CSs and control stimuli may not be the result of differences in their respective conditioning histories. However, since these experiments are relatively easy to carry out there are many different examples to choose from. The defining feature of an opportunistic study is that the experimenter does not actually condition subjects but relies on using subjects' extra-experimental conditioning histories to produced differential responsivity to drug cues.

Conditioned withdrawal

Powell, Gray & Bradley (1993) presented groups of opiate addicts with a slide of somebody injecting the drug, "neutral" cartoon slides, or actual opiate use paraphernalia (injecting or chasing/smoking equipment depending on the subjects' usual route of administration). During the presentation of the drug cues their subjects reported much higher levels of craving than when the neutral cues were present, a finding that is in keeping with all three conditioning models, suggesting that drug CSs would increase the likelihood of drug use. However, of relevance to the conditioned withdrawal model was the finding that subjects also reported much higher levels of dysphoria when the drug cues were present. Subjects also reported higher levels of withdrawal-like symptomatology when the drug cues were present but this difference occurred only in the second of the two cue reactivity tests that were carried out. Although these results support the conditioned withdrawal model, subjects also reported higher levels of drug-positive symptoms during the presence of the drug cues suggesting that responses to drug cues are not exclusively aversive. With alcoholic subjects, studies have also found withdrawal-like responses to the presentation of alcoholic drinks. Kaplan et al. (1985) compared physiological and subjective measures taken from alcoholic and non-alcoholic subjects while they were holding and smelling their favourite alcoholic beverages. Compared with response levels while holding and smelling a "cedar chips" control stimulus, alcoholics had higher heart rates and skin conductance levels, suggesting withdrawal-like responses. However, in this study no differences were found on desire to drink, and it should be noted that increases in skin conductance and heart rate are seen as an effect of alcohol, as well as during alcohol withdrawal (Niaura et al., 1988). This is therefore a study in which the physiological data obtained do not enable the models to be distinguished. A more recent study by Glautier & Drummond (1994) found differences between alcoholic and soft drink cue conditions amongst alcoholics that were more suggestive of a withdrawal-like response. Skin conductance level, self-reported desire to drink, and tension were all higher when the alcoholic drink was present. Anxiety and tension are often seen in alcohol withdrawal.

Conditioned drug-opposite responses and conditioned tolerance

Newlin (1985) carried out two studies in which healthy volunteer subjects drank a non-alcoholic beer which they were told was real beer. Placebo responders who reported intoxication following consumption the non-alcoholic beer, manifested drug-opposite physiological changes consisting of falls in heart rate and skin conductance. Because both the immediate effects of alcohol and alcohol withdrawal are to increase heart rate and skin conductance (Niaura et al., 1988), this study provides support for drug-opposite, rather than withdrawal-like, CRs. However, it is noteworthy that the subjective effects of the placebo were oppositely vectored to the physiological effects. The reports of intoxication used to classify subjects as placebo responders can only really be regarded as drug-like effects, so this may be another example of two apparently different kinds of response being present at the same time. As well as predicting that responses to drug cues should oppose drug effects, Siegel's model suggests that these drug-opposite responses should result in higher tolerance to drug effects when the drug is given in the presence of CSs. A number of studies demonstrate that drugs given in familiar contexts have smaller effects and therefore support this hypothesis. Both Remington, Roberts & Glautier (submitted) and McCusker & Brown (1990) found that alcohol has greater detrimental effects on cognitive and motor skills when it is given in unusual vehicle mixtures and in an unusual context (McCusker & Brown contrasted a daytime office setting with an evening simulated bar). One recent study by Ehrman et al. (1992) involved opiate addicts receiving opiates either through their usual self-injection ritual or via an automatic infusion. The infusion produced larger increases in skin temperature and decreases in heart rate while during the cook-up ritual preceding self-injection heart rate increases and skin temperature falls were seen.

Conditioned drug-like responses

Data from both of the preceding sections can also be adduced in support of the model of drug-like responses to drug CSs. As we have already seen, on measures where withdrawal effects and immediate drug effects are in the same direction any evidence for one model is by default also support for the other. Thus, the Kaplan et al. (1985) and Glautier & Drummond (1994) studies found skin conductance and heart rate responses to alcohol cues which support the conditioned drug-like response model. Also, the Powell, Gray & Bradley (1993) study gives simultaneous support to drug-like and withdrawal-like response models because evidence for both kinds of response was found on different measures. Finally, in the Newlin (1985) study, subjects' reports of intoxication following consumption of a placebo suggest drug-like responses. An additional noteworthy study reported by O'Brien (1976), showed that when opiate addicts injected themselves with saline they apparently experienced a euphoric effect.

Conditioning Experiments

In contrast to opportunistic experiments, conditioning studies manipulate the relationship between cues and drug presentations. By doing so it is hoped that any differences in responses produced by the drug cues can be directly attributed to the fact that the experimenter has exposed subjects to an association between a cue and drug delivery. Therefore, evidence from this kind of study may generally be regarded as higher in internal validity than that from opportunistic studies, provided of course that reasonable controls have been adopted.

Conditioned withdrawal

Although there have now been a number of experimental demonstrations which support the view that withdrawal symptoms can be used as the basis of conditioning, some provide only indirect support for Wikler's theorizing. One widely cited study, Wikler & Pescor (1967, described in Wikler, 1980), involved rats first being made physically dependent on morphine and then transferred to a regimen in which a single high dose was given at the start of each day. This regimen caused the rats to experience a daily cycle of withdrawal which was at a peak immediately before the dose, and at an intermediate stage about 12 hours after dosing. By restricting the movement of the rats to a particular area of the cages during the withdrawal phase it was possible to ensure that these areas of the cage were paired with withdrawal. Tests for conditioning, carried out by placing experimental and control rats in different cage areas, showed that the experimental rats showed more conditioned withdrawal symptoms ("wet dog shakes") than the controls. Thus, these results indicate conditioning of morphine withdrawal symptoms, although they certainly do not unambiguously show that cues present when drugs are ingested are associated with the subsequent adaptive response to the drug dose, as Wikler proposed. Another study, this time with human methadone-maintained addicts, also showed that opiate withdrawal symptoms could be conditioned (O'Brien, 1976). To do this, O'Brien presented subjects with the sound of a tone and a peppermint oil smell immediately before they received an injection of naloxone which precipitated a withdrawal state indicated by symptoms including runny eyes and nose, yawning, gooseflesh, rise in blood pressure, and fall in skin temperature. The pairing of the stimulus complex with the injection was repeated between six and 11 times in order to establish it as a predictor of acute withdrawal. The effect of conditioning was assayed in a test using a saline injection procedure. Self and observer ratings of the subjects' withdrawal severity indicated that responsiveness to the cue complex increased dramatically between a pre-conditioning test and a post-test.

However, in both of these studies the effective US may well have been the drug withdrawal state itself. This is not quite the same as the scheme originally proposed in which a CS paired with an immediate drug effect elicits withdrawal symptoms. In one study by Kelsey, Aranow & Matthews (1990) that kind of evidence was found. Contexts which rats experienced for 1 hour immediately after a morphine injection elicited withdrawal-like symptoms.

Conditioned drug-opposite responses and conditioned tolerance

McCaul, Turkkan & Stitzer (1989) reported an experiment in which they gave alcoholic subjects a dose of alcohol every day for 4 days, before substituting a placebo drink on a fifth test day. A control group experienced the placebo drink on each of the 4 days and also on the fifth test day. For the experimental group, in which the vehicle drink mixture was intended to be a CS for alcohol delivery, there was a fall in heart rate and skin conductance relative to controls following the drink on the test day, evidence for drug-opposite CRs. Also using an alcohol US, Le, Poulos & Cappell (1979) found that rats exhibited hyperthermic responses to a CS for alcohol delivery. Since alcohol's temperature effects are of a biphasic nature (Niaura et al., 1988) this is another piece of evidence in which the predictions of two models do not provide a clear basis for differentiation of the approaches.

Although these findings support Siegel's model they do not, on their own, do full justice to it. This is because, in addition to handling the observation that drug CSs increase drug use motivation by hypothesising the occurrence of drug-opposite CRs, Siegel asserts that these CRs mediate tolerance to a drug's effects. Moreover, since tolerance means that a higher dose of drug is required to produce the same effect it is entirely conceivable that tolerance and drug use would be closely linked. If a conditioning process can mediate drug tolerance, either through drug-opposite CRs or otherwise, it can also influence drug use.

There is now a large body of evidence which shows that tolerance to drug effects is affected by situational factors (see Goudie & Demellweek, 1986; Siegel, 1989, for reviews). For example, Siegel, Hinson & Krank (1978) showed that tolerance to the analgesic effects of morphine was lost if the drug delivery was accompanied by changes in the circumstances of administration. Many other experiments have replicated this basic finding. Using human subjects, Dafters & Anderson (1982) found that changing the context of alcohol delivery resulted in loss of tolerance to the tachycardic effects of alcohol. Similarly, Remington, Roberts & Glautier (submitted) assessed the effect of presenting alcohol to regular beer drinkers in a novel vehicle solution, i.e. in the absence of normal alcohol CSs. Fifteen minutes after drinking, the latter group showed markedly greater impairment of cognitive and motor performance, and more profound subjective measures of intoxication. It should be noted here, however, that opponent processes may not be necessary to explain how conditioning processes may affect drug tolerance. For example, Baker & Tiffany (1985) proposed that a habituation model based on Wagner's (1976) general theoretical account of associative learning provides a better account of the literature on tolerance to drug effects than does Siegel's conditioned opponent model. Thus, evidence for conditioned tolerance does not necessarily lead to support for the model of drug-opposite CRs.

Conditioned drug-like responses

Schwartz & Cunningham (1990) carried out an experiment in which they infused rats with morphine through an indwelling catheter and monitored temperature responses. In one group of rats, the experimental group, the infusion was given 30 seconds after the onset of a light and white noise CS lasting 15 minutes. In the other group, the control group, the drug was given 75 minutes after the offset of the CS. Thus, for the experimental subjects the CS predicted the onset of drug effects whereas for the controls this predictive CS–US contingency was absent. In test sessions the experimental group had the infusion delayed in order to allow the observation of responding to the CS. Evidence for drug-like responses to the CS was found; the morphine infusions produced increases in body temperature and in the group for which the CS was paired with morphine, presentation of the CS also resulted in increases in body temperature. The conditioning experiment (Glautier, Drummond & Remington, 1994) described in the introduction to this chapter can also be taken as supporting evidence for drug-like CRs since alcohol may increase skin conductance. However, as with other examples described these effects may also support other models since the effect of alcohol and the effect of alcohol withdrawal may be iso-directional (Niaura et al., 1988).

DEFICIENCIES OF THE MONISTIC MODELS

Given that there are three accounts of the nature of conditioned responses to drug cues and drug taking, a reasonable question is: which one is correct? Eikelboom & Stewart (1982) suggested that anyone seeking order in this area is immediately faced with a mass of contradictory findings, and even the small number of studies cited so far is sufficient to underline their point. Data from a wide range of sources involving both human and animal subjects can be used either to support or refute each model. Indeed, one may legitimately begin to wonder whether a definitive evaluation is possible. If the models just described can all garner some support under some circumstances then perhaps the goal of parsimony is better served by adopting a different strategy in an attempt to bring order to the data. One possible solution stems from an examination of the more general classical conditioning literature. This shows that the problem of CR form is a central one for learning theorists to which there is no complete solution as yet (Mackintosh, 1983). What is clear, however, is that CRs can take a range of different forms, and that several factors play an important role in determining the particular CR seen in any given circumstance. In particular, the characteristics of both the US and of the CS have been identified as important determinants of the nature of the CR.

With reference to the role of the US, we will argue that such stimuli are complex events inducing changes in multiple response systems, each of which has particular physiological characteristics and pharmacological sensitivities. Moreover, the effects generated in any response system are temporally extended, and may be biphasic. Unless these characteristics are taken into account, any attempt to define the form of CR with direct reference to unconditioned drug effects (e.g. drug-like, drug-opposite, withdrawal-like) is unlikely to be a valid generalization simply because of its limited conceptualization of the UR, if for no other reason. In addition, we will show there is now good evidence that the stimulus properties of any particular CS can themselves affect the form of CR. Further complexity is added by the fact that there will often be multiple stimuli that can potentially function as drug CSs in any given drug use situation.

Unconditioned Stimulus Characteristics

The US used in any particular conditioning preparation critically affects both the form of the UR and the CR. For example, a food US elicits a

UR of salivation, while a footshock US elicits leg flexion; when CSs for food and footshock occur, salivation and leg flexion are elicited. However, this description of events is certainly a gross oversimplification of reality because the effects of food and footshock USs are a great deal more complex. This becomes clear when the effects of the US are examined more closely. Mackintosh summarizes the situation like this:

> Most USs have both sensory and affective properties and elicit compensatory reactions as well as discrete, overt URs. It is implausible to suppose that a CS paired with a US is associated with one of these attributes or consequences to the exclusion of all others. (Mackintosh, 1983, p. 65)

The central point being made here is that USs have multiple attributes and affect multiple response systems. For example, footshock does not simply elicit leg flexion, it also induces anxiety, bodily withdrawal from the source of the shock, heart rate and skin conductance change, and a multitude of other forms of behavioural variation. Therefore, if one attempts to describe a CR with reference to the effects of a US it is necessary to be quite specific about which of its attributes are being referenced. In terms of drug conditioning, the unconditioned effects of alcohol, to take a common example, include vasodilatation, increased heart rate, changes in hedonic state such as feelings of well-being and disinhibition, marked changes in social behaviour, and decrements in performance on psychomotor and cognitive tasks. Similarly, the effects of morphine include amongst others hyperthermia, changes in hedonic state such as feelings of well-being and contentedness, and sedation. Add to this the fact that many drugs have actions that change over quite an extended period of time and a picture of great complexity emerges. To make matters worse, specific attributes of the UR may be particularly salient to particular forms of CS (Mackintosh, 1983). For example, a punctate visual CS such as the illumination of a small light bulb can be approached or withdrawn from, but the possibility of directed locomotor activity is precluded if a diffuse auditory CS such as a tone is used.

Multiple response domains

The evidence presented so far on the form of CRs to drug CSs has rather arbitrarily been selected from the wide range of possibilities that are available. The theories of Wikler, Stewart, and Siegel are pitched at a very general level and it is clear that their predictions have been tested in behavioural, subjective and physiological domains. Little has been made of the fact that some experiments have reported behavioural data, some have reported on the subjective state of subjects on the basis of self-report questionnaires, others have gathered physiological data, whereas still others have simultaneously gathered data from more than one domain. As the foregoing discussion suggests, however, our current understanding of classical conditioning processes makes it less than appropriate to evaluate Wikler's, Stewart's, and Siegel's theories while ignoring the response domains from which the data have been obtained.

But are the standard accounts of CR form supported more consistently if response systems in the physiological, behavioural, and subjective domains are considered separately? It seems clear that they are not. For example, conflicting evidence can easily be found in the subjective and physiological domains as the data already presented show. When behavioural measures such as activity level or "wet dog shakes" are considered, a similarly inconsistent picture emerges. Again, it seems as though different kinds of drug effect can be conditioned under different circumstances. For example, Wikler & Pescor (1967) were able to condition morphine withdrawal symptoms ("wet dog shakes"), whereas Siegel (1975[2]) has shown hyperalgesic responses (drug-opposite) to cues for morphine. At least one kind of behavioural measure should show more consistency. Where measures of motivation to drink, such as rate of consumption of an alcoholic drink (e.g. Hodgson, Rankin & Stockwell, 1979), are concerned, the position should be clear. All theories predict that presentation of drug cues should increase the likelihood of drug use but of course such a measure fails to discriminate between accounts of CR form. Moreover, in some limiting cases, even this assumption fails. For example, a cue for a self-administered drug may elicit avoidance behaviours, and any drug of abuse can function as an aversive as well as an appetitive stimulus. In particular, when an organism has never previously experienced a drug's effects, an aversion to it, and to cues for its delivery, can be formed (Hunt & Amit, 1987). In addition, high doses of drugs of abuse can be aversive even to regular users because of their toxic or incapacitating action (Griffiths, Bigelow & Henningfield, 1980).

Individual response system attributes

Given the diversity even within the broad response domains just discussed, perhaps it is to be expected that uniform results have not been obtained. Considering only the physiological domain with its many systems (heart rate, skin conductance, muscular control systems, and so on) arranged in complex and interactive ways, it might begin to seem unlikely that we will be able to make useful generalizations even at one level and unfortunately, this seems to be the case. Moreover, if even a single physiological response system is analysed in detail there are still apparent variations in response directionality when different conditioning preparations are used. For example, in a conditioning study using two different drugs (atropine and morphine), which have opposite unconditioned effects on salivation, Rush, Pearson & Lang (1970) found that CSs for both drugs produced increases in salivation. Thus, even within the context of a single response system (salivation) it is possible for drug CRs to take on different forms by comparison to their URs (i.e. drug-like or drug-opposite responding). Rush, Pearson & Lang (1970) also found that the tachycardia UR produced by both drugs only occurred as a CR to a morphine-paired CS. They explained their results by pointing to the fact that atropine and morphine have different physiological sites of action, atropine acting largely in the periphery and morphine largely centrally. It was proposed that because peripheral drug effects are less easily conditionable, it was not possible to obtain heart rate conditioning with an atropine US.

Rush, Pearson and Lang's suggestion that the site of a drug's action in the nervous system plays an important role in conditioning of drug effects has remained influential. Eikelboom & Stewart (1982) have gone on to develop this line of argument by suggesting that a drug has two possible sites of action, either on the afferent (input) side of the central nervous system (CNS) or on the efferent (output) side. Only when a drug acts on the afferent side, however, is its observed action properly called a UR. For example, if a hypothetical drug acted to increase baroreceptor[3] output through direct action on the baroreceptor, the observed fall in blood pressure that would follow increased output would constitute a "genuine" UR. Therefore, any CS for the drug would produce a fall in blood pressure, resembling the observed UR. On the other hand, if the drug increased baroreceptor output indirectly, for example by producing peripheral vasoconstriction, then the drug's initial observed action (increased blood pressure) is not a UR. Rather, the later homeostatic adjustment to the increased blood pressure is the UR. According to Eikelboom & Stewart, the CR will always resemble the true UR, but it will not resemble any initial peripheral effect of a drug. Thus, the model suggests that failure to consider the different sites of drug action can result in mislabelling the observed responses to drugs, thereby creating the impression of CRs opposing or resembling URs. So, according to Eikelboom & Stewart's approach, the determination of whether responses to CSs really resemble or oppose the responses to USs requires detailed physiological knowledge of the way that a drug exerts its observed effects. This approach to the form of response to drug cues would predict that different response directionality would appear when different response systems were considered depending on where in the regulatory feedback loop the drug had its action. As we will see later, however, an explanation of this kind can still encounter difficulties if different CSs for the same US produce different effects.

Temporal characteristics of unconditioned responses

In addition to the need to consider the site of action of the US, some theorists (e.g. Solomon & Corbit, 1973, 1974; Wagner, 1981) emphasized the importance of the temporal parameters of US action. Such considerations seem particularly important with drug US which, unlike a sudden noise or a pellet of food, is temporally extended for minutes or hours. Solomon & Corbit (1973, 1974) proposed that the repeated presentation of any stimulus which has significant consequences for an organism (either as a reward or punishment) will eventually result in a reduced response to that stimulus. For example, a strongly aversive stimulus such as confronting a parachute jump for the first time may initially produce a variety of responses including heart rate accelerations, incoherent vocalization, and gross physical movements, which collectively might be said to reflect "terror". Following repeated exposure, the situation induces smaller responses, perhaps merely reflecting "anxiety". Moreover, with experience, feelings of pleasure and well-being are often reported when a jump is completed (Epstein, 1967). Solomon considered the temporal dynamics of opiate use to be similar, although the polarity of the emotions induced are reversed. Early in a career of use, the addict experiences a "rush" or an intensely pleasurable sensation, but after repeated exposure the injection merely results in "relief" or normality and, as this feeling dissipates, aversive withdrawal sets in.

In order to explain these phenomena, Solomon & Corbit propose that all reinforcing and aversive stimuli tend to have biphasic effects. An initial effect, termed an "α process", elicits in turn a second effect, termed a "β process", which acts to oppose or counteract the initial homeostatic disturbance. Because α and β processes oppose one another, the net response to any stimulus is reduced when the β process is strong. Furthermore, whereas α processes are fixed and determined by the physical properties of the stimulus applied and the nervous system of the organism concerned, the β process is strengthened as a result of experience with stimuli which produce α processes. Initially, the β process has a small magnitude, a long latency to onset, and a short duration. After repeated production of the α state, the ensuing β process has a larger magnitude, a shorter latency to onset and a longer duration. The net effects of any stimulus will therefore have smaller magnitudes, shorter latencies to peaks and shorter durations as a result of the development of β processes. The β process was argued to be a "slave" process in that its initial elicitation and growth is dependent entirely upon the occurrence of an α process.

Wagner (1981) applied some of the ideas found in Solomon & Corbit's opponent process theory in the SOP memorial model (Sometimes Opponent Process or Standard Operating Procedures of memory) of classical conditioning. In SOP, responses that are elicited by stimuli arise as a result of the activation of a cognitive representation of the stimulus. The cognitive system is conceptualized as a large collection of nodes, and representation of a stimulus involves the activity of a group of these nodes. Any particular node may be in one of three states, inactive (I), active type 1 (A1), or active type 2 (A2). When a US is presented, its nodes will initially move to state A1 and then gradually decay over time to state A2 before finally becoming inactive again. The sum of activity in A1 and A2 states determines the behavioural output. Thus, when the A1 and A2 states have opposite behavioural effects the UR will have a biphasic form, as often occurs with strongly hedonic stimuli.

The significance of this for the present discussion is that the SOP model assumes that a CS can only ever trigger the A2 representation of the US, and the CR will therefore sometimes oppose the UR. In particular, if the later action of a US is opposite in sign to the initial action (reflecting an opposition of A1 and A2 states), then the CR will oppose the initial UR. Paletta & Wagner (1986) carried out studies in which they applied SOP theory to predicting the form of CRs to CSs for morphine in rats. They reported that the unconditioned locomotor effects of morphine had a time course in which an immediate sedative action was followed by an increase in activity, whereas its analgesic effect was monophasic. After the conditioning phase of their study, they found that morphine-paired contexts elicited increases in activity, evidence for a compensatory response, whereas these contexts had no effect on pain sensitivity. Although these studies support SOP theory, it is possible for the apparently biphasic action of morphine on activity measures to have been the result of two independent drug actions (e.g. sedation and activation) each with a different time course, and Paletta & Wagner acknowledge this point. Their experiments nevertheless show the value of an approach in which different kinds of CR are explicitly allowed for and attempt to take into account something of the complexity of UR form.

Conditioned Stimulus Characteristics

The second main component of any conditioning preparation is the CS itself. However, although the CS is typically a weaker stimulus than the

US its effects on the outcome of conditioning cannot be ignored. Already we have noted that different kinds of CS may be especially suited to forming associations with different kinds of US (or different kinds of US attribute) but it is necessary to recognize that CS form may have its own direct impact on the form of CR.

In one investigation of this topic, Holland (1977) used two groups of rats. In one group, L+, a light was established as a cue for food, and a tone was unpaired. For the other group, T+, the reverse contingencies applied. Over the course of conditioning, a number of differences in response to light and tone developed. Presentation of the tone CS+ resulted in a general increase in activity, as measured by stabilometer counts, but light CS+ did not. However, this difference in activity did not mean that the light was ineffective as a CS+. Detailed observation of the rats' behaviours during CS+ presentation revealed that L+ rats showed increases in rearing and magazine behaviours during the CS (which presumably did not affect the stabilometer) whereas T+ rats showed increasing amounts of head jerking during the CS (which presumably did affect the stabilometer).

In further explorations of this effect, Holland (1977, 1980) showed that it was not the case that different CSs result in different amounts of learning about the USs, as in research on prepared associations (Garcia & Koelling, 1966). Rather, responding to the CS appears to be a joint function of the nature of the orienting response (OR) unconditionally elicited by the CS, and of the responses elicited by the US. Furthermore, responses occurring earlier in the CS–US interval are influenced more by the form of the CS than responses later in the CS–US interval, which are related to imminent US arrival and are similar for different kinds of CS.

The implications of these findings for our consideration of response to drug cues are clear and have already received investigation. There are a large number of potential CSs for drug delivery in the natural setting (perhaps with different characteristic for different drugs, e.g. beer odours and pub sounds for drinkers, venepuncture and syringes for heroin addicts) and many of these can be used in experimental settings. If the choice of CS varies arbitrarily from one study to the next, the results of investigations may appear capricious. On the other hand, considering the nature of the CS may bring some order to seemingly meaningless data. For example, Table 2.1 summarizes a number of studies of alcohol cue reactivity involving human subjects. The data are grouped according to the nature of the CS used, specifically whether subjects consumed (upper half) or did not consume (lower half) the placebo drink. These data suggest that decreases in indices of arousal, skin conductance and

Table 2.1   Summary of studies examining physiological responses to alcohol cues with human subjects. Studies in the top half of the table, marked D, involved subjects actually consuming drinks whereas the studies in the bottom half of the table, marked H, involved subjects merely holding drink stimuli

Authors		SC	IBI	SAL	FPV	PTT	TEM
McCaul et al. (1989)	D	−	+				0
Newlin (1985)	D	−	+		0	0	0
Macfarlane & White (1989)	D		+				
Staiger & White (1988)[1]	D		+				0
Newlin (1986)	D		0		0	−	0
Newlin (1989)[2]	D		−				0
McCusker & Brown (1990)	D		+				
Turkkan et al. (1989)[3]	H	+	−				−
Kaplan et al. (1985)	H	+	−	+			
Kaplan et al. (1983)	H	+	0				0
Pomerleau et al. (1983)	H	0	0	+			
Monti et al. (1987)	H			+			

[1] Responses to drink cues alone were increase in heart rate.
[2] Female subjects used.
[3] A taste of drink included.
+, Increase; −, decrease; 0, no result, blank, not measured; D, drink consumed; H, drink held; SC, skin conductance; IBI, interbeat interval; SAL, salivation; FPV, finger pulse volume; PTT, pulse transit time; TEM, temperature.
Reproduced from Glautier, Drummond & Remington (1992) with permission of Springer-Verlag.

heart rate (i.e. increasing interbeat interval) are seen when drinks are consumed (i.e. held, smelled, tasted and swallowed), whereas increases tend to occur when drinks are merely held and smelled. However, none of these studies directly compared the effect of consumption versus non-consumption on the direction of responding to alcohol-related cues. Therefore, Glautier, Drummond & Remington (1992) carried out a study designed to investigate the effect of presenting different elements of the stimulus complex making up an alcohol CS. Using alcohol-free beer as a putative CS, two groups of non-dependent drinkers were presented with the kind of alcohol cues that either typically precede drinking (e.g. the sight and smell of beer) or that co-arise with drinking (e.g. sight, smell and taste). Two control groups of subjects saw, smelled and tasted, or simply saw and smelled, peppermint-flavoured water. Physiological, subjective and behavioural responses were measured and the main results of this study supported the view that the differences in the directionality of cue reactivity may be affected by the modality of the alcohol-related cues. The pattern of results was consistent with those in Table

2.1; holding tended to produce relative increases in skin conductance and vasoconstriction and falls in pleasure ratings whereas drinking produced the opposite pattern.

Although it is possible that the mechanism by which these results were obtained was similar to that elucidated by Holland, it is by no means the only possible way for different kinds of cue to influence response form. At present, in many published studies of alcohol cue responsivity, there is an implicit assumption that differences between drug and control stimuli arise because of differences in the conditioning histories of the cues (see Glautier and Tiffany, this volume, Chapter 4). Holland's research indicates that the conditioning process may interact with the unconditioned responding elicited by the events used as CSs to produce the observed CRs. Fortunately, however, there are a few examples of the way in which CS form influences CR form in drug conditioning paradigms. Staiger & White (1988) carried out a conditioning experiment using an alcohol US and human subjects, and Eikelboom & Stewart (1981) carried out a conditioning study with rats using morphine as US. Staiger & White's study found that context (room cues) CSs produced responses opposite in direction to those produced by the local drink CSs (vehicle mixture). On the other hand, Eikelboom & Stewart found opposite responses depending upon whether or not temporal CSs (time of day) or environmental CSs (room cues) were used.

The last two sections have considered the role of the US and CS in relation to the form of CR. Unconditioned stimuli have multiple effects in different response domains, but even considering response domains separately still yields conflicting data on CR form. Indeed, even if a single response system such as salivation is considered, CRs may have different forms in relation to US effects when different drug USs are used. Part of the explanation for this kind of effect may relate to the physiological site of action of different drugs. According to Eikelboom & Stewart (1982), some drugs may act on the afferent arm of the CNS, in which case their effects may properly be considered as stimuli; CRs to CSs for these drugs will resemble the observed effect of the drug. Other drugs, however, may act on the efferent arm of the CNS and so should not be regarded as stimuli; CRs to CSs for these drugs will appear to oppose the effects of the drug. Furthermore, we have seen that drug effects change over time and may be biphasic in nature. It may be the case that typically the later action of the drug is conditioned, and if this opposes the initial effect then drug-opposite CRs will be seen. However, even taking into account the physiological site of drug action and information on its time course, we still could not predict CR form of a single response system as long as CS form remains unspecified. It may be difficult to make sense of comparisons between experiments that have even quite small differences in procedure. In the case of experiments using human subjects, an additional problem is encountered when cues are presented in a way that disrupts the normal course of drug consumption. Subjects' expectancy of drug consumption and the special demand characteristics imposed by the unusual procedure may render results difficult to interpret.

CONCLUDING REMARKS

Early in this chapter we questioned the possibility that simple models of CR form would be adequate to explain the data. They have not proved to be so. As a corollary, simple models of the motivational functions of cues are also inadequate. For example, to suggest that responses to drug cues resemble drug withdrawal states is an oversimplification; likewise, to suggest that conditioned withdrawal symptoms underlie the motivational functions of drug cues is also an oversimplification. It may certainly be argued that sometimes CRs do resemble withdrawal states, and that it is in these circumstances that cues will increase drug use motivation. Thus, a conditioned withdrawal model of drug use motivation could be sustained in the face of conflicting data on CR form by arguing that only conditioned withdrawal had a motivational impact. Watering the argument down still further by allowing different kinds of CR and different kinds of motivational function would cease to make this a conditioned withdrawal model at all. The approach being advocated here is that CRs have different forms and many factors contribute to the outcomes that are observed. However, an additional proposition is that the form of responses to a cue will not in general allow a prediction of its effect on drug seeking behaviours.

The earlier consideration of responses to cues in different response domains makes the point that the theories of conditioned withdrawal, conditioned drug-opposite responses, and conditioned drug-like responses are no better supported in one domain or another. However, the fact that there are multiple response systems which can be conditioned needs to be taken into account and, if anything, makes it seem even less likely that a single theory of response form could succeed. To illustrate this, it is only necessary to imagine that all experiments looking at physiological responses to alcohol cues had obtained the same finding, e.g. that alcohol cues inevitably produced increases in skin conductance. Would this contain any necessary implication for subjective or behavioural systems? In other words, is it possible to assess the psychological or behavioural effects of cue presentation on the basis of an assessment of the physiological state? The answer must be a resounding no. Unfortunately the enterprise of predicting the state of one response system on the basis of another is fraught with difficulty since there is a universe of events with unknown size which, for example, could produce changes in drinking behaviour (Caccioppo & Tassinary, 1990).

This is not to argue that behavioural, subjective and physiological states are independent of one another. In fact, they are inextricably intertwined and mutually interdependent. They can be seen as different levels at which analyses can be pitched (Cacioppo & Tassinary, 1990), but the implications of an analysis in one domain for events in another are far from straightforward. For example, in the analysis of neurosis, the term "desynchrony" has been applied in acknowledgement of the difficulties in mapping relationships between behaviour, subjective state, and physiology (Hodgson & Rachman, 1974; Rachman, 1978). Tiffany (1990) has assessed the interrelationships amongst response domains during presentation of drug cues, and shown that in many studies correlations between cue reactivity measures and behavioural measures of drinking were not reported or were rather low. Although long-term research aims must be to develop models which can integrate data from different domains, this should not discourage investigation of individual domains. In fact, a focus on one domain or another can be seen as an important simplifying step and may provide a way into an otherwise complicated and difficult area. However, given the central social importance of drug seeking behaviour itself, it might be argued on pragmatic grounds alone that the effects of presentation of drug cues on drug seeking should be a priority area. Provided that other factors influencing drug taking, such as deprivation or experimental demand characteristics, are carefully controlled, drug seeking behaviour is the most direct assay of the motivational effects of cue presentation. By making it the variable of interest, the need to make difficult connections between CR form, inferred motivational state, and then drug taking is avoided.

NOTES

1. In practice, a drinks counterbalancing procedure was used. Half the subjects experienced the same colour/flavour/alcohol/soft drink assignments described whereas the arrangements were reversed for the other half.

2. This is a controversial finding as there have been a number of failures to replicate (e.g. see Goudie & Demellweek, 1986).

3. Baroreceptors are stretch receptors sited on the walls of arteries. As blood

pressure increases the artery wall is stretched causing a change in the output of the receptor which will co-vary with changes in blood pressure.

REFERENCES

Baker, T.B. & Tiffany, S.T. (1985). Morphine tolerance as habituation. *Psychological Review*, **92**, 78–108.

Cacioppo, J.T. & Tassinary, L.G. (1990). Psychophysiology and psychophysiological inference. In J.T. Cacciopo & L.G. Tassinary (Eds), *Principles of Psychophysiology: Physical, Social and Inferential Elements*. New York: Cambridge University Press.

Dafters, R. & Anderson, G. (1982). Conditioned tolerance to the tachycardia effect of ethanol in humans. *Psychopharmacology*, **78**, 365–367.

Drummond, D.C., Cooper, T. & Glautier, S.P. (1990). Conditioned learning in alcohol dependence: implications for cue exposure treatment. *British Journal of Addiction*, **85**, 725–743.

Edwards, G. (1990). Withdrawal symptoms and alcohol dependence: fruitful mysteries. *British Journal of Addiction*, **85**, 447–461.

Ehrman, R., Ternes, J., O'Brien, C.P. & McLellan, A.T. (1992). Conditioned tolerance in human opiate addicts. *Psychopharmacology*, **108**, 218–224.

Eikelboom, R. & Stewart, J. (1981). Temporal and environmental cues in conditioned hypothermia and hyperthermia associated with morphine. *Psychopharmacology*, **72**, 147–153.

Eikelboom, R. & Stewart, J. (1982). Conditioning of drug induced physiological responses, *Psychological Review*, **89**, 507–528.

Epstein, S.M. (1967). Towards a unified theory of anxiety. In B.A. Maher (Ed.), *Progress in Experimental Personality Research*, Vol. 4. New York: Academic Press.

Garcia, J. & Koelling, R.A. (1966). The relation of cue to consequence in avoidance learning. *Psychonomic Science*, **4**, 123–124.

Glautier, S. & Drummond, D.C. (1994). Alcohol dependence and cue reactivity. *Journal of Studies on Alcohol*, **55**, 224–229.

Glautier, S., Drummond, D.C. & Remington, B. (1992). Different drink cues elicit different physiological responses in non-dependent drinkers. *Psychopharmacology*, **106**, 550–554.

Glautier, S., Drummond, D.C. & Remington, B. (1994). Alcohol as an unconditioned stimulus in human classical conditioning. *Psychopharmacology*, **116**, 360–368.

Goldberg, S.P., Woods, J.H. & Schuster, C.R. (1969) Morphine: conditioned increases in self administration in rhesus monkeys. *Science*, **166**, 1306–1307.

Goudie, A.J. & Demellweek, C. (1986). Conditioning factors in drug tolerance. In S.R. Goldberg & I.P. Stolerman (Eds), *Behavioural Analysis of Drug Dependence*. London: Academic Press.

Griffiths, R.R., Bigelow, G.E. & Henningfield, J.E. (1980). Similarities in animal and human drug taking behaviour. In N.K. Mello (Ed.), *Advances in Substance Abuse*, Vol. 1. Greenwich: JAI Press.

Hodgson, R. & Rachman, S. (1974). II. Desynchrony in measures of fear. *Behaviour Research and Therapy*, **12**, 319–326.

Hodgson, R., Rankin, H. & Stockwell, T. (1979). Alcohol dependence and the priming effect. *Behaviour Research and Therapy*, **17**, 397–387.

Holland, P.C. (1977). Conditioned stimulus as a determinant of the form of the pavlovian conditioned response. *Journal of Experimental Psychology: Animal Behaviour Processes*, **3**, 77–104.

Holland, P.C. (1980). Influence of visual conditioned stimulus characteristics on form of pavlovian appetitive conditioned responding in rats. *Journal of Experimental Psychology: Animal Behaviour Processes*, **6**, 81–97.

Hunt, T. & Amit, Z. (1987). Conditioned taste aversion induced by self administered drugs: paradox revisited. *Neuroscience and Biobehavioural Reviews*, **11**, 107–130.

Kaplan, R.F., Cooney, N.L., Baker, L.H., Gillespie, R.A., Meyer, R.E. & Pomerleau, O.F. (1985). Reactivity to alcohol related cues: physiological and subjective responses in alcoholics and non-problem drinkers. *Journal of Studies on Alcohol*, **46**, 267–272.

Kelsey, J.E., Aranow, J.S. & Matthews, R.T. (1990). Context-specific morphine withdrawal in rats: duration and effects of clonidine. *Behavioural Neuroscience*, **104**, 704–710.

Le, A.D., Poulos, C.X. & Cappell, H. (1979). Conditioned tolerance to the hyperthermic effects of ethyl alcohol. *Science*, **206**, 1109–1110.

Mackintosh, N.J. (1983). *Conditioning and Associative Learning*. Oxford: Clarendon Press.

McCaul, M.E., Turkkan, J.S. & Stitzer, M.L. (1989). Conditioned opponent responses: placebo challenge in alcoholic subjects. *Alcoholism: Clinical and Experimental Research*, **13**, 631–635.

McCusker, C.G. & Brown, K. (1990). Alcohol predictive cues enhance tolerance to and precipitate craving for alcohol in social drinkers. *Journal of Studies on Alcohol*, **51**, 494–499.

Newlin, D.B. (1985). The antagonistic placebo response to alcohol cues. *Alcoholism: Clinical and Experimental Research*, **9**, 411–416.

Niaura, R.S., Rohsenow, D.J., Binkoff, J.A., Monti, P.M., Pedraza, M. & Abrams, D.B. (1988). *Journal of Abnormal Psychology*, **97**, 133–152.

O'Brien, C.P. (1976). Experimental analysis of conditioning factors in human narcotic addiction. *Pharmacological Reviews*, **27**, 533–543.

Paletta, M.S. & Wagner, A.R. (1986). Development of context specific tolerance to morphine: support for a dual process interpretation. *Behavioural Neuroscience*, **100**, 611–623.

Poulos, C.X., Hinson, R.E. & Siegel, S. (1981). The role of Pavlovian processes in drug tolerance and dependence: implications for treatment. *Addictive Behaviours*, **6**, 205–211.

Powell, J., Gray, J. & Bradley, B.P. (1993). Subjective craving for opiates: evaluation of a cue exposure protocol for use with detoxified opiate addicts. *British Journal of Clinical Psychology*, **32**, 39–53.

Powell, J., Gray, J.A., Bradley, B.P., Kasvikis, Y., Strang, J., Barrat, L. & Marks, I. (1990). The effects of exposure to drug-related cues in detoxified opiate addicts: a theoretical review and some new data. *Addictive Behaviours*, **15**, 339–345.

Rachman, S.J. (1978). *Fear and Courage*. San Francisco: Freeman.

Remington, B., Roberts, P. & Glautier, S. (submitted). Effects of drink familiarity on alcohol tolerance. *Addictive Behaviours*.

Rescorla, R.A. (1988). Pavlovian conditioning: it's not what you think it is. *American Psychologist*, **43**, 151–160.

Rush, M.L., Pearson, L. & Lang, W.J. (1970). Conditional autonomic responses induced in dogs by atropine and morphine. *European Journal of Pharmacology*, **11**, 22–28.

Schull, J. (1979). A conditioned opponent theory of Pavlovian conditioning and habituation. In G.H. Bower (Ed.), *The Psychology of Learning and Motivation*, Vol. 13, pp. 57–90. New York: Academic Press.

Schwartz, K.S. & Cunningham, C.L. (1990). Conditioned stimulus control of morphine hyperthermia. *Psychopharmacology*, **101**, 77–84.

Siegel, S. (1975). Evidence from rats that morphine tolerance is a learned response. *Journal of Comparative and Physiological Psychology*, **89**, 498–506.

Siegel, S. (1989). Pharmacological conditioning and drug effects. In A.J. Goudie & M.W. Emmett-Oglesby (Eds), *Psychoactive Drugs: Tolerance and Sensitisation*. Clifton, NJ: Humana Press.

Siegel, S., Hinson, R.E. & Krank, M.D. (1978). The role of predrug signals in morphine analgesic tolerance: support for a pavlovian conditioning model of tolerance. *Journal of Experimental Psychology: Animal Behaviour Processes*, **4**, 188–196.

Solomon, R.L. & Corbit, J.D. (1973). An opponent-process theory of motivation: II. Cigarette addiction. *Journal of Abnormal Psychology*, **81**, 158–171.

Solomon, R.L. & Corbit, J.D. (1974). An opponent-process theory of motivation: I. Temporal dynamics of affect. *Psychological Review*, **81**, 119–145.

Staiger, P.K. & White, J.M. (1988). Conditioned alcohol-like and alcohol-opposite responses in humans. *Psychopharmacology*, **95**, 87–91.

Stewart, J., de Wit, H. & Eikelboom, R. (1984). Role of unconditioned and conditioned drug effects in the self-administration of opiates and stimulants. *Psychological Review*, **91**, 251–268.

Tiffany, S.T. (1990). A cognitive model of drug urges and drug-use behaviour: the role of automatic and non-automatic processes. *Psychological Review*, **97**, 147–168.

Wagner, A.R. (1976). Priming in STM: an information processing mechanism for self-generated or retrieval-generated depression in performance. In T.J. Tighe & R.N. Leaton (Eds), *Habituation: Perspectives from Child Development, Animal Behaviour and Neurophysiology*. Hillsdale, NJ: Erlbaum.

Wagner, A.R. (1981). SOP: a model of automatic memory processing in animal behaviour. In N.E. Spear & R.R. Miller (Eds), *Information Processing in Animals: Memory Mechanisms*. Hillsdale, NJ: Laurence Erlbaum Associates.

Wikler, A. (1948). Recent progress in research on the neurophysiologic basis of morphine addiction. *American Journal of Psychiatry*, **105**, 329–338.

Wikler, A. (1980). *Opioid Dependence: Mechanisms and Treatments*. New York: Plenum Press.

Wikler, A. & Pescor, F.T. (1967). Classical conditioning of a morphine abstinence phenomenon, reinforcement of opioid drinking behaviour and relapse in morphine addicted rats. *Psychopharmacologia*, **10**, 255–284.

Wise, R.A. & Bozarth, M.A. (1987). A psychomotor stimulant theory of addiction. *Psychological Review*, **94**, 469–492.

CHAPTER 3

Potential functions of classical conditioning in drug addiction

Stephen T. Tiffany*

Addicts presented with drug-relevant stimuli in cue reactivity studies often display increases in drug craving, changes in patterns of autonomic responding, and, in some cases, alterations in their drug-seeking behavior (Baker, Morse & Sherman, 1987; Niaura et al., 1988; Rohsenow et al., 1990). Since its inception, interpretations of the cue reactivity paradigm have been derived primarily from the framework of classical conditioning. During a history of drug use, certain stimuli, such as environmental contexts or drug paraphernalia, reliably accompany drug administration. It is typically assumed that these stimuli, by virtue of their pairing with the drug unconditioned stimulus (US), become conditioned stimuli (CSs) capable of eliciting conditioned responses (CRs). From this perspective, addicts' reactions to presentations of drug-paired stimuli in a cue reactivity study are considered CRs.

If situations and objects associated with drug administration acquire the properties of conditioned stimuli, then it is of considerable theoretical and clinical import to evaluate the functional significance of classical conditioning in drug-dependence disorders. That is, what role might conditioned stimuli play in either the development or maintenance of self-administration of drugs? This question is part of the more general issue addressed by animal-learning theorists of the possible influence of classical conditioning on instrumental performance of all sorts. Curiously, important developments from this literature have had, at best, only limited influence on conceptualizations of the function of classical conditioning in addictive disorders. In fact, some currently popular versions of how classical processes might affect drug taking invoke views of classical/instrumental interactions regarded as outmoded in the learning literature for over two decades.

*Purdue University, West Lafayette, Indiana, USA

Addictive Behaviour: Cue Exposure Theory and Practice.
Edited by D.C. Drummond, S.T. Tiffany, S. Glautier and B. Remington.
© 1995 John Wiley & Sons Ltd.

This chapter will provide an overview and evaluation of classical conditioning theories of addictive behavior. Although the primary focus will be on the relevant human data, the models will also be examined from the standpoint of applicable animal research on drug conditioning and the status of the general conditioning theory represented in each model. This review will not be exhaustive, but should provide readers unfamiliar with this literature sufficient background for more extensive study. The chapter will conclude with a consideration of alternate hypotheses regarding the potential role of classical conditioning in drug use, views compatible with contemporary theorizing in animal learning but not currently represented in conditioning theories of addictive behavior. No new theory of classical conditioning and drug addiction will be advanced in this chapter. However, these proposals may promote the development of an elaborated view of the possible functions of classical conditioning in drug taking and suggest new approaches to the study and interpretation of cue reactivity phenomena.

CONDITIONED WITHDRAWAL MODELS OF DRUG ADDICTION

The first and most influential model of conditioning and drug addiction was offered by Wikler (1948) who proposed that environmental stimuli paired with drug withdrawal become CSs capable of eliciting conditioned withdrawal reactions. Wikler contended that abstinent heroin addicts, confronted with situations where they had previously undergone drug withdrawal, would be motivated to seek out and use heroin (i.e. relapse) to alleviate these aversive conditioned withdrawal reactions. A more recent model of addiction (Poulos, Hinson & Siegel, 1981; Siegel, 1983) hypothesizes that withdrawal-like effects are elicited by the presentation of cues associated, not with drug withdrawal, but with the administration of drugs. This theory is based on the hypothesis (Siegel, 1975) that stimuli reliably paired with drug delivery elicit conditioned responses that are opposite in direction to, or compensatory for, the direct or unconditioned effects of the drug. These conditioned responses are believed to be responsible for conditioned tolerance effects when the addict is under the influence of drug and conditioned withdrawal-like effects when the addict is not drugged. The motivational impact of these conditioned responses is presumed to be the same as Wikler's (1948) model of conditioned withdrawal; the abstinent addict will find these responses aversive and will relapse in an effort to alleviate them.[1]

The compensatory response model and the conditioned withdrawal model of addiction differ only with regard to the nature of the cues, drug-paired or withdrawal-paired, that should elicit conditioned withdrawal effects. As any given bout of drug use in the experienced addict may pair the same stimuli with both drug administration and drug withdrawal, this distinction may be difficult to discern in the addict's world (Tiffany & Baker, 1986).[2] This difficulty notwithstanding, the compensatory response model appears to offer some conceptual and empirical advantages over Wikler's (1948) conditioned withdrawal model of addiction. First, there is considerable evidence that drug tolerance can be strongly influenced by classical conditioning (see reviews by Baker & Tiffany, 1985; Goudie & Demellweek, 1986; Siegel, 1983). In contrast, the animal evidence in favor of conditioned withdrawal effects is less extensive (e.g. Goldberg & Schuster, 1970; Wikler & Pescor, 1967). Second, there is, as of yet, little indication from the addictions literature that environments exclusively paired with drug withdrawal, e.g. detoxification centers, act as strong elicitors of conditioned, withdrawal-like reactions or craving (McAuliffe et al., 1986). Finally, the compensatory response model allows for the acquisition of conditioned responses over the course of an addict's history of drug use, in that each drug administration constitutes a conditioning trial. In Wikler's model, conditioning begins only after the addict has sufficient exposure to the drug to develop an unconditioned withdrawal syndrome. Thus, the compensatory response model provides a mechanism for the maintenance of drug use operating even in the early phases of drug self-administration. Moreover, it is difficult to conceive how, in Wikler's model, environmental stimuli paired with drug administration could ever acquire strong associative control over withdrawal reactions. Until unconditioned withdrawal was firmly established, addicts would have extensive, unreinforced exposure to environmental stimuli that, when subsequently paired with withdrawal, are to operate as conditioned stimuli. These unreinforced exposures would constitute a latent inhibition procedure severely restricting the ability of these stimuli to sustain conditioning (e.g. Lubow, 1989; Tiffany & Baker, 1981).

The hypothesis that relief of an aversive withdrawal state reinforces drug taking represents a specific instance of a more general two-process model of aversively motivated instrumental behavior (e.g. Mowrer, 1947; Schlosberg, 1937). Two-process theories argue that learning to avoid aversive USs relies on both classical and instrumental conditioning. For example, in a signalled avoidance task, animals are presented some cue, such as a brief tone, that reliably precedes the administration of an aversive event, such as electric shock. If the task is structured so the animal can engage in some response to avoid or terminate the shock after the signal is presented, it will readily learn to avoid shock. Mowrer (1947) hypothesized that the signal, by virtue of its pairing with the aversive US becomes, through classical conditioning, a CS that elicits aversive visceral CRs. These CRs constitute a conditioned fear reaction serving to increase the vigor of avoidance behavior. If an avoidance response leads to the termination or degradation of the fear-eliciting CS, the subsequent reduction of the conditioned fear reinforces avoidance behavior. According to this model, avoidance learning really represents learning to escape from the aversive CS. As applied to addiction, the acquisition of drug-administration behavior can be conceptualized as escape learning, which is reinforced through the alleviation of conditioned withdrawal (see Figure 3.1).

Evaluation of the Role of Conditioned Withdrawal in Addiction

Conditioned withdrawal models of addiction have had several strong advocates over the past four decades (O'Brien et al., 1988; Poulos, Hinson & Siegel, 1981; Siegel, 1983, 1989; Wikler, 1948, 1972, 1974), and the reader may wish to consult reviews by these proponents for a full discussion of the evidence in support of this approach. However, a full consideration of the relevant data presents serious challenges for the hypothesis that drug-paired stimuli exert their influence on drug self-

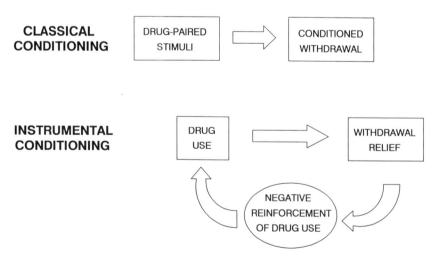

Figure 3.1 Conditioned withdrawal model of addiction.

administration primarily through conditioned withdrawal effects. The evidence can be summarized as follows.

Empirical status of conditioned compensatory responses

As predicted by Siegel (1975), many instances of drug tolerance appear to reflect the operation of classical conditioning, yet there is substantially less support for the assumption that these conditioned tolerance effects are necessarily subserved by conditioned compensatory or withdrawal-like responses (e.g. Baker & Tiffany, 1985; Goudie & Demellweek, 1986). For example, we have had considerable success demonstrating conditioned tolerance to the analgesic effects of morphine (Cepeda-Benito & Tiffany, 1992; Tiffany, Drobes & Cepeda-Benito, 1992; Tiffany & Maude-Griffin, 1988; Tiffany, Maude-Griffin & Drobes, 1991), but have never obtained any indication of conditioned hyper-responsivity to a painful stimulus when animals expecting morphine were given a placebo in a drug-paired context (Maude-Griffin & Tiffany, 1989; Tiffany et al., 1983; Tiffany, Cepeda-Benito & Sanderson, 1994).

Several proponents of compensatory response models of conditioned tolerance, acknowledging the elusive nature of conditioned compensatory responses, have suggested that a number of factors may obscure their detection in placebo tests (Hinson, Poulos & Cappell, 1982; King, Bouton & Musty, 1987; Poulos & Cappell, 1991; Siegel, 1989). As one possibility, the interoceptive effects produced by the drug may constitute a critical component of the CS complex producing conditioned tolerance effects (Greeley et al., 1984; cf. Cepeda-Benito & Tiffany, 1993). Animals given a placebo in a drug-paired context may not display a compensatory response because they are not given the full CS (i.e. the drug effects as well as the context) responsible for conditioned responding. This and similar explanations for failures to obtain indications of compensatory responding in non-drugged animals may preserve the compensatory response theory of drug tolerance. But, if drug delivery is necessary for the generation of compensatory responding, then the value of this model for explaining an addict's motivation to use drugs is diminished. How could a drug-paired context motivate any instance of drug use if the addict had to first use the drug before the aversive conditioned response could be generated?

Autonomic responses to drug cues

The conditioned withdrawal models of addiction assume that the patterns of physiology elicited by presentations of drug-paired cues to addicts should resemble the autonomic physiology of withdrawal. There are examples of withdrawal-like physiological reactions from some research (e.g. Childress et al., 1988), but, on balance, most cue reactivity studies provide little foundation for the assumption that autonomic responses elicited by drug-paired cues mimic drug withdrawal (see reviews by Niaura et al., 1988; Rohsenow et al., 1990). Conditioned withdrawal models also predict that the autonomic responses elicited by drug-paired stimuli should be strongly associated with measures of drug-use behavior obtained under the same stimulus conditions. Tiffany (1990) summarized all the cue reactivity studies that allowed for an evaluation of associations between cue-elicited physiological measures and various indices of drug use. Across the studies reviewed, only three of the 37 correlation coefficients between these two types of measures were significant, and even these few significant correlations provided scant evidence for a strong, direct relationship between physiological responses and drug use.

Drug withdrawal and relapse

Conditioned withdrawal models assume that relapse is driven by the elicitation of withdrawal-like effects by drug-related cues. Evidence from follow-up studies of addicts who have undergone treatment indicates that relapse is more frequent in the presence of stimuli or situations strongly associated with previous drug use, but addicts who have relapsed rarely report that they experienced withdrawal reactions just prior to their reinitiation of drug use (e.g. Marlatt & Gordon, 1980).

Motivational properties of drug-paired stimuli

A central tenet of the two-process model of avoidance is that stimuli paired with aversive events acquire aversive properties. If true, then it should be possible to demonstrate that animals will be reinforced for engaging in behavior that terminates the presentation of a classically conditioned aversive stimulus. This prediction has received considerable empirical support (see review by Levis, 1989). Similarly, the conditioned withdrawal approach to addiction supposes drug-paired stimuli acquire aversive properties. Therefore, termination of these stimuli should act as a reinforcer. One implication of this assumption is, if escape from a drug-paired context is reinforcing, addicts should readily learn to avoid or leave environments associated with their previous drug use. Although this prediction has not been tested directly, clinical lore suggests that, rather than avoid drug-paired stimuli, addicts readily seek out situations and contexts associated with their previous drug use. Complementary evidence from animal investigations shows drug-paired stimuli do not uniformly elicit aversive effects. For example, if given a choice, animals tend to show preferences, not aversions, for environments paired with opiates, cocaine, amphetamine, and alcohol (see review by Robinson & Berridge, 1993).

Contemporary status of two-process avoidance theory

The version of avoidance learning adopted by most withdrawal-based conceptualizations of addiction, Mowrer's (1947) two-process theory, is regarded by many reviewers as an inadequate account of aversively motivated behavior (e.g. Mineka, 1979, 1985; Hulse, Egeth & Deese, 1980; Domjan, 1993; Gray, 1975; Rescorla & Solomon, 1967; cf. Levis, 1989). Some of the difficulties faced by Mowrer's theory may not confront a conditioned withdrawal model of addiction. For example, Mowrer's (1947) theory has been challenged by findings that, once established, avoidance behavior tends to be extremely persistent, but fear responses to the CS, which supposedly maintain that behavior, may decline over training (e.g. Kamin, Brimer & Black, 1963). It is not surprising that fear responses might weaken under these circumstances; successful avoidance responding will prevent the delivery of the US in the presence of the CS. Such a situation should promote extinction. Yet, the extinction of fear poses problems for the supposition that reductions in conditioned fear sustain escape from the CS. This dilemma may not confront a two-process account of addiction. Conditioned withdrawal theories posit that organisms learn a response, drug use, that functions directly to ameliorate the aversive consequences of withdrawal CRs. Such behavior would allow for a continued pairing of the drug US with contextual stimuli; thus conditioning to the CSs would be maintained over the course of drug use.

One shortcoming of the two-process avoidance model with particular relevance for conditioned withdrawal models is the lack of evidence of a close correspondence between specific responses elicited by fear-conditioned stimuli and avoidance responding (Rescorla & Solomon, 1967). As noted above, the absence of a clear relationship between cue-elicited physiological responses and drug self-administration poses similar difficulties for the conditioned withdrawal model of addiction.

Conclusion

The hypothesis that responses to drug-paired stimuli reflected conditioned withdrawal effects and that these effects were central to the maintenance of drug administration in the addict was seminal in the development of the cue reactivity paradigm. The influence of this view was derived from its theoretically plausible account of both the situational specificity of relapse and the occurrence of relapse long after the abatement of unconditioned withdrawal effects. The theory was also compatible with the traditional emphasis in the addictions field on drug withdrawal as the primary motivational process subserving drug use. The legitimacy of this approach was further bolstered by its association with a two-process theory of avoidance learning that had dominated the study of fear behavior through the 1950s, but was supplanted by modern theories of classical–instrumental interactions in the 1960s (e.g. Rescorla & Solomon, 1967). Now, nearly half a century after its introduction, the conditioned withdrawal model (Wikler, 1948; Poulos, Hinson & Siegel, 1981), confronted with the plethora of negative results described above, no longer provides a compelling account of drug addiction.[3]

THE CONDITIONED INCENTIVE MODEL OF DRUG ADDICTION

Stewart, de Wit & Eikelboom (1984) proposed a model of drug addiction that offered a perspective on the motivational significance of drug-paired stimuli differing substantially from the withdrawal-based view. This theory diverged from the conditioned withdrawal approaches in two fundamental ways. First, it hypothesized that stimuli associated with drug delivery became positive incentives that drove drug use. Thus, in this model, the appetitive features of drugs rather than drug withdrawal determined drug self-administration. Second, this model relied on a pure classical conditioning approach or single process theory of learning. According to this theory, conditioned incentive stimuli elicit a motivational state that directly primes drug-taking behavior. In contrast, the conditioned withdrawal model invokes two forms of learning, classically conditioned withdrawal and the instrumental acquisition of drug-use behaviors reinforced through relief of withdrawal.

The conditioned incentive model hypothesizes that all drugs of abuse act on common neural substrates to generate positive appetitive states maintaining drug use. Environmental stimuli paired with administration of drugs become conditioned stimuli that activate neural states mimicking the direct appetitive effects of drugs. These environmental stimuli function as conditioned incentives that, when presented, impel the organism to engage in drug use (see Figure 3.2). The model proposes that, in addition to conditioned incentive effects, drug-paired stimuli

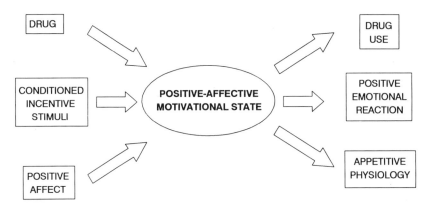

Figure 3.2 Conditioned incentive model of addiction (Stewart, de Wit & Eikelboom, 1984).

might have other influences on drug-seeking behavior. Stewart, de Wit & Eikelboom (1984) hypothesized these CSs might elicit conditioned physiological responses that enhance the direct, unconditioned incentive value of drugs. If so, drug administration would invoke a more intense positive affective state when it occurs in an environment associated with previous drug use. Any enhancement of the unconditioned incentive properties of the drug would increase the likelihood of readministration of the drug in those circumstances. Drug-paired stimuli might also elicit conditioned emotional states similar to the positive affective reactions triggered by the drug itself. These conditioned emotional states can presumably prime further drug use.

Although Stewart, de Wit & Eikelboom's (1984) model incorporated concepts derived from a wide range of motivational research and theory, this framework was derived principally from Bindra's (1972, 1974, 1978) conceptualization of incentive motivation. According to Bindra, motivated behavior arises from an interaction of organismic states and incentive stimuli. He hypothesized that motivationally relevant stimuli are invested with unconditioned incentive properties such that their presentation produces constellations of appetitive or aversive reactions. The sight, taste and odor of food, for example, will elicit approach and consummatory behaviors. The central motivational state of the organism will have a selective excitatory or inhibitory influence on the incentive properties of stimuli. These influences work to regulate the animal's transactions with stimuli relevant to its current motivational state. For instance, a food-deprived animal will be more likely to approach and eat food than a non-deprived animal. Central motivational states also mediate the production of patterns of autonomic physiology appropriate to the particular state. A hungry animal, for example, might salivate. Incentive stimuli also excite or activate central motivational states; the presentation of a palatable food to a sated animal should elicit salivation and eating (e.g. Weingarten, 1983).

From Bindra's perspective, hedonic stimuli control behavior through their primary and conditioned motivational incentive properties. Bindra's (1972, 1974, 1978) approach to learning rests entirely on stimulus–stimulus associations or classical conditioning. Thus, this model rejects the notion that instrumental performance represents a form of learning distinct from classical conditioning. Hedonically neutral stimuli, if paired with the presentation of primary incentives, become, through the operation of classical conditioning, secondary incentives. These acquired incentive stimuli are able to activate central motivational states and will elicit the range of responses normally controlled by primary incentives. In essence, the animal will treat conditioned incentives as if they were primary incentives. The phenomenon of autoshaping (Brown & Jenkins, 1968) can be conceptualized as a dramatic example of incentive learning. If a response key is lighted each time food is delivered to a pigeon, the animal will begin to peck at the lighted key. The topography of the pecking behavior suggests that the bird is attempting to eat the key.

Evaluation of Role of Conditioned Incentives in Addiction

Stewart, de Wit & Eikelboom (1984) presented considerable evidence that the positive incentive effects of drugs motivate drug-use behavior. The strongest support comes from the clear demonstrations that animals will readily self-administer drugs of abuse. These findings illustrate that addictive drugs can function as powerful positive reinforcers, effects not mediated through drug withdrawal mechanisms. Furthermore, as described earlier, place conditioning studies show animals will display a preference for environments paired with drug administration. Such results suggest drug-paired contexts become secondary incentives that motivate approach behaviors. Stewart, de Wit & Eikelboom (1984) also reviewed research showing that small doses of drugs administered noncontingently could reinstate drug-taking behavior after extinction training. Similarly, stimuli previously paired with the administration of drugs could also reinstate drug self-administration following extinction training. The incentive motivational interpretation of these demonstrations is that presentation of either a priming dose of a drug or stimuli paired with drugs can reactivate an appetitive motivational state facilitating drug-seeking behavior. Finally, some reviewers of the cue reactivity literature have noted that the patterns of autonomic responses observed in addicts presented with drug-paired stimuli appear more similar to the activating or stimulating effects of drugs than to the physiology of drug withdrawal (e.g. Niaura et al., 1988; Rohsenow et al., 1990). This depiction of the autonomic data is more compatible with an appetitive or positive incentive characterization of drug conditioning than with a withdrawal-based account.

The conditioned incentive model offered by Stewart, de Wit & Eikelboom (1984) has had a powerful influence on research and theory on addictive behavior. It has been applied with increasing frequency in interpretations of the results of many cue reactivity studies (e.g. Rohsenow et al., 1990), and several other theorists have incorporated ideas regarding the motivational influence of positive incentive effects of drugs into their accounts of drug addiction (e.g. Baker, Morse & Sherman, 1987; Markou, Weiss, Gold et al., 1993; Niaura et al., 1988; Robinson & Berridge, 1993; Wise, 1988). However, despite its numerous successes, the model faces conceptual and empirical difficulties and does not, in its present form, provide a complete account of several major features of cue reactivity phenomena. Some of the problems that confront this model are as follows.

Specification of core motivational processes

Much of the evidence adduced in favor of an incentive motivational view of addiction comes from demonstrations that animals will learn to engage in behaviors that result in the administration of drugs. These findings are consistent with Stewart, de Wit & Eikelboom's (1984) model, but they are equally compatible with any conceptualization of addiction that drugs motivate self-administration through their positively reinforcing properties (e.g. Brady, 1991; Johanson, 1990; Schuster & Thompson, 1969; Wise, 1988; Young & Herling, 1986). Showing that drugs act as primary positive reinforcers certainly challenges the view that withdrawal processes account for all drug motivation, but does not compel the adoption of an appetitive motivational explanation for those effects. Some reviewers have conflated evidence for the positively reinforcing effects of drugs as support for an incentive motivational model of positive reinforcement (e.g. Markou et al., 1993). Unfortunately, the incentive model described by Stewart, de Wit & Eikelboom (1984) is not sufficiently articulated to permit that model to be distinguished from any other theory that also assigns positive reinforcement a central role in addictive behavior.

A related problem is that the theory's core motivational mechanisms are not clearly stipulated. At various points, Stewart, de Wit & Eikelboom (1984) contend that positively affective motivational states, appetitive motivational processes, positive reinforcement, euphoria, and craving are responsible for drug use. This assortment of terms makes it difficult to specify the kinds of data critical to the evaluation of the motivational features of the model. For example, should ratings of craving, drug-induced euphoria, and positive affect all be tightly coupled to measures of drug use in addicts? More generally, it seems implausible that the various systems represented by this diversity of terms all derive from the activation of a unidimensional motivational mechanism.

Application of incentive motivation model to drug addiction

The heuristic value of Bindra's (1972, 1974, 1978) incentive motivation framework for studying drug self-administration seems restricted by important differences between drug reinforcers and conventional appetitive reinforcers. Unlike natural incentives such as food and water, the reinforcing effects of drugs cannot be manipulated in non-dependent organisms through the induction of some deprivation condition. Furthermore, drugs have no naturally occurring primary incentive stimuli unconditionally eliciting drug-specific approach and consummatory behaviors. Stewart, de Wit & Eikelboom (1984) acknowledge these differences but provide no discussion of how Bindra's conceptualization of incentive motivation and incentive learning might have to be modified to accommodate the idiosyncrasies of the drug-use situation. For example, Bindra (1978) details how the building of representations of contingencies between natural incentives and conditioned stimuli could provide the sole basis of learning. Without a primary incentive stimulus, it is not immediately apparent that the rules of learning governing the acquisition of drug self-administration would be the same as those posited by Bindra for more conventional reinforcers.

Status of single-process learning theory

Most contemporary animal-learning theorists accept the idea that classical contingencies may contribute to the acquisition and control of instrumental behavior, but few, if any, are willing to endorse the relatively radical proposition embedded in Bindra's theorizing and adopted by Stewart, de Wit & Eikelboom (1984), that *all* instrumental learning can be reduced to stimulus–stimulus associations or classical conditioning (see reviews by Domjan, 1993; Mackintosh, 1983; Rescorla, 1988; and commentaries following Bindra's (1978) theoretical review). The conceptual and empirical difficulties confronting a single-process theory of conventional incentives may be compounded in a single-process model of drug reinforcement, which, as noted above, would be forced to assemble a theory of learning without the benefit of naturally occurring incentives or deprivation states.

Interpretations of autonomic responses

Some reviewers of the cue reactivity literature have concluded that patterns of autonomic responses elicited by drug-paired cues seem more consistent with an appetitive motivational model than a withdrawal-based approach to drug conditioning (Niaura et al., 1983; Rohsenow et al., 1990). Whereas addicts often do display autonomic activation in the presence of drug stimuli, such as increased heart rate and skin conductance, the unequivocal attribution of these responses to the mobilization of an appetitive motivational system is complicated by two factors. First, a unique autonomic profile of appetitive motivational or positive affective states has not been, and likely will not be, established. Research on the psychophysiology of emotion shows that, whereas particular emotional states might display some characteristic patterns of autonomic responding, the general categories of positive and negative affect cannot be distinguished on the basis of autonomic physiology (Levenson, 1992).

Second, the constellation of autonomic responses found in many cue reactivity studies is compatible with several alternative explanations. Consider the finding of increased heart rate during imagery of smoking-relevant stimuli (Drobes & Tiffany, 1994; Maude-Griffin & Tiffany, 1994; Tiffany & Hakenewerth, 1991). Although this might reflect the activation of a positively affective motivational state, it might also be due to preparation for physical activity (Obrist et al., 1970), cognitive effort associated with urge processing (Tiffany, 1990), defensive responding (Baker et al., 1984), negative affect provoked by frustration over not being able to smoke, or even isodirectional conditioning of nicotine-induced tachycardia (Stephens, 1977). These diverse possibilities illustrate how an autonomic response to a drug-relevant stimulus cannot be construed unambiguously as a specific indicant of a given psychological process.

Relationships between autonomic responses and craving or drug use

If the physiological responses observed in cue reactivity studies are due to the activation of an appetitive motivational state, then these responses should be associated with other indices of this state including craving report, positive affect, and drug use. Examination of the cue reactivity literature reveals little indication of strong or even consistently moderate relationships between cue-specific autonomic reactions and craving or mood report (Tiffany, 1988, 1990). As reviewed in the section on withdrawal-based models, there is even less indication of any meaningful association between cue-specific physiological reactions and measures of drug-use behavior (Tiffany, 1990).

Affective qualities of cue reactions

A pivotal prediction of the incentive motivational model is that presentation of drug-paired stimuli to addicts should elicit a positive affective reaction. Stewart, de Wit & Eikelboom (1984) cite Levine (1974) and O'Brien and his colleagues (O'Brien et al., 1974) as showing that intravenous drug users derive pleasure and report euphoria when they inject themselves with a placebo under conditions previously associated with drug delivery. Actually, no formal measures or statistical analyses of affect or euphoria were reported in any of these studies. Consequently, they provide no documented support for the claim that drug-paired cues invariably elicit positive affect. Even the informal descriptions of the results suggested that, when they occurred, pleasurable effects from a placebo injection were typically weak and transient (O'Brien, 1976; O'Brien et al., 1974, 1980).

More rigorous evaluations of affective reactions to presentations of drug-paired stimuli provide little support for the prediction that these cues consistently induce positive affect. For example, a meta-analysis of research using the alcohol balanced placebo design showed that expectancy of alcohol consumption had no overall significant impact on mood report (Hull & Bond, 1986). Cue reactivity studies with cigarette smokers have found repeatedly that presentations of smoking-relevant stimuli generally enhance negative mood and/or decrease positive mood (e.g. Burton, Drobes & Tiffany, 1992; Cepeda-Benito & Tiffany, 1994; Drobes & Tiffany, 1994; Maude-Griffin & Tiffany, 1994; Elash, Tiffany & Vrana, 1994; Tiffany & Drobes, 1990). These findings directly contradict a major premise of the incentive motivational model of addiction.

Conclusion

Like the conditioned withdrawal model, the incentive motivational theory invoked classical conditioning to explain the situational specificity of relapse as well as the occurrence of relapse long after the cessation of drug use. This theory has, by and large, supplanted the conditioned withdrawal model as the dominant animal-learning approach to drug motivation (Markou et al., 1993; Robinson & Berridge, 1993). The ascendancy of this model can be attributed to a number of factors. First, its publication helped crystallize a growing conviction in the addictions field that the positively reinforcing effects of drugs contributed to drug dependence disorders. Second, unlike a radical behavioral conceptualization of positive reinforcement, this theory offered a psychological model of drug use that fused both motivational and learning mechanisms into a conceptually rich account of drug reward. Finally, the acceptance of the model was further aided by its connection to complementary research on the physiology and pharmacology of appetitive reward systems (see review by Robinson & Berridge, 1993).

However, the incentive motivational model faces conceptual and empirical shortcomings similar to those confronting the conditioned withdrawal theory of addiction. In both cases, data from the cue reactivity literature do not conform to the models' characterizations of how addicts should respond to drug-paired stimuli. Moreover, the learning theories embraced by either model cannot be considered representative of major trends in contemporary learning theory. This chapter will conclude with a sampling of modern views of the potential role of classical conditioning in instrumental performance, and discuss the application of these concepts to the cue reactivity paradigm.

CONTEMPORARY PERSPECTIVES ON CLASSICAL/INSTRUMENTAL INTERACTIONS

Modern Two-process Theory

Mowrer (1947) presumed that specific, overt conditioned responses were responsible for the instrumental acquisition of escape behavior. Rescorla & Solomon (1967) concluded that the available evidence provided little support for this theory of avoidance and proposed an alternative framework, which has come to be known as modern two-process theory. This approach hypothesizes that conditioned stimuli can elicit a central emotional state functioning to motivate or modulate instrumental behavior. The emotional state would be positive or negative depending on whether the reinforcer was, respectively, aversive or appetitive. In the case of an appetitive task, in which an animal is trained to respond for a reinforcer such as food, a stimulus that reliably precedes the presentation of the reinforcer becomes a CS. Over training, this CS elicits a central emotional state that would function to increase instrumental responding for food. Conditioned emotional states of the same valence as the emotional state evoked by the instrumental reinforcer should augment responding in the instrumental task. If the states are of opposite valence, instrumental performance should be inhibited. For example, presentation of a stimulus previously paired with shock during a food-motivated instrumental task should decrease instrumental responding (e.g. Kamin & Brimer, 1963). Modern two-process theory has received scant attention in the addictions literature and, with one exception, has not been applied systematically to cue-reactivity research. Drummond, Cooper & Glautier (1990) used the theory to hypothesize how, in cue-exposure treatments, extinction of drug-paired stimuli might, paradoxically, increase rather than decrease drug-use behavior.

In contrast to Mowrer's (1947) conceptualization, the conditioned emotional state envisioned by modern two-process theory is not necessary for instrumental performance; it merely functions to modulate instrumental behavior. Furthermore, as the emotional state has no specific, fixed representation in overt responses, this theory eschews research that attempts to identify particular constellations of conditioned responses elicited by CS presentations. The research strategy suggested by this theory is the transfer-of-control experiment (Rescorla & Solomon, 1967), which examines the impact of classically conditioned stimuli on instrumental performance. Research using this paradigm has provided considerable evidence that one factor involved in classical–instrumental interactions is the central emotional state evoked by classically conditioned stimuli (Domjan, 1993). Transfer-of-control experiments might be useful for investigating whether the affective state evoked in addicts by presentations of drug-paired stimuli is essentially appetitive or aversive. If drug-predictive cues elicit an appetitive emotional state, then presentation of these cues during a non-drug appetitive task, such as working for monetary reward, should enhance performance. These same cues should decrease responding on an aversively motivated task. In contrast, if drug cues establish an aversive emotional reaction, their presentation should disrupt performance on an appetitive task and enhance performance on an aversive task.

Reinforcer-specific Expectancies

Some transfer-of-control experiments indicate, in addition to general central emotional states, stimuli paired with reinforcers in instrumental tasks may elicit expectancies for specific reward outcomes (e.g. Baxter & Zamble, 1982; Kruse et al., 1983; Peterson & Trapold, 1980). Baxter & Zamble (1982) demonstrated that a CS paired with electrical brain stimulation increased instrumental responding for brain stimulation reward but did not augment responding for food. Instrumental responding for food reward was increased, however, by the presentation of a CS that had been paired with food delivery. These results suggest conditioned stimuli may establish expectancies for particular rewards, and these expectancies may influence instrumental responding for that reinforcer.

The potential influence of reward-specific expectancies on drug use might be particularly relevant for investigations of poly-drug abusers. For example, alcoholics who are also heavy smokers could be required to work on instrumental tasks reinforced by either alcohol or nicotine. If drug-paired cues establish reward-specific expectancies, then the presentation of smoking-related stimuli during the tasks should specifically enhance responding for nicotine, whereas alcohol-related cues should specifically enhance instrumental performance for alcohol.

Hierarchical Relationships in Instrumental Learning

From a two-process perspective, reinforcers or outcomes (Os) are involved in the formation of two kinds of associations during instrumental learning. First, they establish the link between stimuli (Ss) and responses (Rs). In addition to S–R associations, instrumental tasks allow for the formation of classically conditioned associations between antecedent stimuli and outcomes (S–O associations). All the models considered so far in this chapter assumed that these S–O associations were responsible for the influence of classical conditioning over instrumental performance. There is also evidence that organisms may acquire associations between specific responses and outcomes (e.g. Colwill & Rescorla, 1986), and it has been hypothesized that these R–O associations serve as critical mediators in instrumental learning (e.g. Bolles, 1972; Colwill, 1993; Mackintosh & Dickinson, 1979; Rescorla, 1991).

Other research and theory on the associative structure of instrumental learning suggests the operation of even more complex relationships in the modulation of instrumental performance. Several researchers have noted that instrumental learning involves a conditional relationship between stimuli and outcomes such that the stimulus is followed by a reinforcer only if the animal performs a response. These relations can be represented by the hierarchical notation, S(R–O), which can be translated as stating that, under certain stimulus conditions, particular responses produce specific outcomes. It has been hypothesized that instrumental performance is controlled, not through S–R associations, but by S(R–O) associations. That is, R–O associations are activated conditionally through the presentation of S (e.g. Colwill & Rescorla, 1990; Jenkins, 1985; Rescorla, 1990, 1991; Skinner, 1938).

The hypothesized hierarchical control of instrumental learning has parallels in research on facilitation or occasion setting in classical conditioning (e.g. Holland, 1985; Rescorla, 1985; Ross, 1983). In this research, contingencies can be established such that one stimulus, the occasion setter, can serve as cue for the pairing of another stimulus with a US. This conditional association could be represented in the hierarchical notation, S(CS–US), which is similar to the S(R–O) relation posited for hierarchical control of instrumental learning. Occasion setters do not seem to have the usual excitatory properties of traditional CSs, but appear to operate by activating the CS–US relation. For example, non-reinforced exposure to an occasion setter has no impact on its ability to modulate conditioned responding to the CS (e.g. Rescorla, 1985; Ross, 1983). Some researchers have suggested that occasion setters in classical conditioning and discriminative stimuli in instrumental conditioning represent the operation of comparable processes (e.g. Davidson, Aparicio & Rescorla, 1988).

A consideration of potential hierarchical relations between setting events and response–outcome associations may be particularly relevant for studying the influence of drug-paired stimuli on drug use. A hierarchical conceptualization of instrumental learning suggests, along with the other conditioning theories discussed in this section, that the functional significance of drug-paired stimuli could not be exposed through an examination of responses generated by presentations of those cues. Hierarchical influences are best revealed through transfer-of-control and related experimental designs (e.g. Rescorla, 1991).

The possibility that drug-paired stimuli might regulate drug self-administration through their activation of response–drug associations also has ramifications for cue-exposure treatments of addiction. If stimulus-specific hierarchical relations control drug use, then cue-exposure treatments involving non-reinforced exposures to drug-relevant stimuli are not likely to be effective. In the absence of the opportunity to engage in the drug-use response, non-reinforced exposure to the drug cues would have no impact on the response–drug association. This extinction treatment would only work if the addict engaged in non-reinforced drug use in the presence of drug-predictive stimuli.[4]

SUMMARY

A broader consideration of the routes through which classical processes might modify or regulate instrumental performance has important implications for the conduct and interpretation of cue reactivity research. The traditional view of classical conditioning represented in many studies of cue reactivity emphasizes the functional consequences of the overt responses elicited by presentations of drug-paired stimuli. These conditioning theories stress the role of either conditioned withdrawal or conditioned drug excitatory effects as central to the maintenance of drug use in the addict. The research strategy promulgated by these interpretations naturally focuses on identifying specific conditioned responses that serve to mediate drug taking. In contrast, modern learning theories tend to emphasize that observed conditioned responses may only index, or be ancillary to, conditioned central states regulating instrumental behavior. These approaches suggest drug-paired stimuli would elicit classically conditioned central states that might have a profound influence on drug taking, but may not be rigidly fixed to particular constellations of conditioned responses. Thus, these views would not attribute any functional significance to overt, cue-specific reactions to drug-paired stimuli. Instead, they favor research that attempts more directly to identify the influences of conditioned states on drug taking. Contemporary theories of learning offer a rich array of concepts and procedures for investigating the impact of drug-paired stimuli on drug-use behavior. Cue reactivity research could benefit considerably from a systematic exploration of these ideas.

ACKNOWLEDGEMENTS

Preparation of this chapter was facilitated by a research grant (RO1 DAO4050) from the National Institute on Drug Abuse. Kristine Tiffany, Antonio Cepeda-Benito, Susan Barton, Brian Carter, Celeste Elash and Lisa Sanderson provided useful comments on drafts of this chapter. John Capaldi, Terry Davidson and Peter Urcuioli helped clarify some of the ideas presented in this chapter, and Peggy Treece assisted in the preparation of the manuscript.

NOTES

1. The process by which conditioned compensatory responses are translated into drug use has not been clearly specified by Siegel and his colleagues. For example, Poulos, Hinson & Siegel (1981) discuss the possibility that conditioned withdrawal effects are somehow transformed into urges and cravings that, in turn, precipitate relapse. Siegel (1983) speculated that conditioned compensatory responses are ameliorated by drug use, thus producing relapse. Because Wikler's views on the role of conditioned withdrawal in the precipitation of relapse figure so prominently in all their discussions of this topic (Poulos, Hinson & Siegel, 1981; Siegel, 1983, 1989), it seems reasonable to adopt a two-process interpretation of the compensatory response model of addiction.

2. A careful reading of Wikler's statements on this issue indicates that his approach may be more similar to the compensatory response model than has been generally depicted (e.g. Rohsenow et al., 1990). Wikler (1948, 1974) proposed that, over the course of repeated administration of an opiate, the unconditioned response to the drug was transformed from an agonistic effect into a withdrawal reaction. Thus, in the experienced addict, stimuli accompanying drug administration would elicit classically conditioned withdrawal effects. From this perspective, both Wikler (1948) and the compensatory response model posit that stimuli paired with drug administration produce conditioned withdrawal.

3. Conditioned tolerance may foster the development of addictive behavior in ways other than through conditioned withdrawal. For example, development of tolerance to the positively reinforcing properties of a drug would impel the administration of higher doses in order to maintain the same level of reinforcing effect. Similarly, tolerance to negative side effects of a drug, e.g. nausea or dysphoria, would remove barriers to escalation of drug use (Tiffany & Baker, 1986). It is likely that, in the early stages of use, an addict's drug exposures are widely spaced. Although this type of drug-use regimen would not be conducive to the development of non-associative tolerance (Baker & Tiffany, 1985), conditioned tolerance processes could easily bridge the interval between administrations and contribute to an escalation in the amount and frequency of use.

4. The argument that mere non-reinforced exposure to drug-related contexts and drug paraphernalia may not be particularly effective in extinguishing drug-use behavior is not unique to a hierarchical perspective on instrumental learning. Contemporary learning theory offers a variety of reasons why extinction may fail under these circumstances (e.g. Bouton & Swartzentruber, 1991).

REFERENCES

Baker, T.B. & Tiffany, S.T. (1985). Morphine tolerance as habituation. *Psychological Review*, **92**, 78–108.

Baker, T.B., Cannon, D.S., Tiffany, S.T. & Gino, A. (1984). Cardiac response as an index of the effect of aversion therapy. *Behaviour Research and Therapy*, **22**, 403–411.

Baker, T.B., Morse, E. & Sherman, J.E. (1987). The motivation to use drugs: a psychobiological analysis of urges. In P.C. Rivers (Ed.), *The Nebraska Symposium on Motivation: Alcohol Use and Abuse*. Lincoln: University of Nebraska Press, pp. 257–323.

Baxter, D.J. & Zamble, E. (1982). Reinforcer and response specificity in appetitive transfer of control. *Animal Learning and Behavior*, **10**, 201–210.

Bindra, D. (1972). A unified account of classical conditioning and operant training. In H.B. Abraham & W.F. Prokasy (Eds), *Classical Conditioning II: Current Research and Theory*, pp. 453–481. New York: Appleton-Century-Crofts.

Bindra, D. (1974). A motivational view of learning, performance, and behavior modification. *Psychological Review*, **8**, 199–213.

Bindra, D. (1978). How adaptive behavior is produced: A perceptual–motivational alternative to response-reinforcement. *Behavioral and Brain Sciences*, **1**, 41–91.

Bolles, R.C. (1972). Reinforcement, expectancy, and learning. *Psychological Review*, **79**, 394–409.

Bouton, M.E. & Swartzentruber, D. (1991). Sources of relapse after extinction in Pavlovian and instrumental learning. *Clinical Psychology Review*, **11**, 123–140.

Brady, J.V. (1991). Animal models for assessing drugs of abuse. *Neuroscience and Biobehavioral Reviews*, **15** (1), 35–43.

Brown, P.L. & Jenkins, H.M. (1968). Auto-shaping the pigeon's key peck. *Journal of the Experimental Analysis of Behavior*, **11**, 1–8.

Burton, S.M., Drobes, D.J. & Tiffany S.T. (1992). The manipulation of mood and smoking urges through imagery: evaluation of facial EMG activity. Paper presented at the annual meeting of the Midwestern Psychological Association, Chicago.

Cepeda-Benito, A. & Tiffany, S.T. (1992). Effect of the number of conditioning sessions on the development of associative tolerance to morphine. *Psychopharmacology*, **109**, 172–176.

Cepeda-Benito, A. & Tiffany, S.T. (1993). Morphine as a cue in associative tolerance to morphine's analgesic effects. *Pharmacology Biochemistry and Behavior*, **46**, 149–152.

Cepeda-Benito, A. & Tiffany, S.T. (1994). The use of a dual-task procedure for the assessment of cognitive effort associated with smoking urges. Manuscript submitted for publication.

Childress, A.R., McLellan, A.T., Ehrman, R. & O'Brien, C.P. (1988). Classically conditioned responses in opioid and cocaine dependence: a role in relapse. In B.A. Ray (Ed.), *Learning Factors in Substance Abuse*, National Institute on Drug Abuse Monograph 84, pp. 25–43. Washington, DC: US Government Printing Office.

Colwill, R.M. (1993). An associative analysis of instrumental learning. *Current Directions in Psychological Science*, **2**, 111–116.

Colwill, R.M. & Rescorla, R.A. (1986). Associative structures in instrumental learning. In G.H. Bower (Ed.), *The Psychology of Learning and Motivation*, Vol. 20, pp. 55–104. San Diego: Academic Press.

Colwill, R.M. & Rescorla, R.A. (1990). Evidence for the hierarchical structure of instrumental learning. *Animal Learning and Behavior*, **18**, 71–82.

Davidson, T.L., Aparicio, J. & Rescorla, R.A. (1988). Transfer between Pavlovian facilitators and instrumental discriminative stimuli. *Animal Learning and Behavior*, **16**, 285–291.

Domjan, M. (1993). *The Principles of Learning and Behavior*, 3rd edn. Pacific Grove: Brooks/Cole.

Drobes, D.J. & Tiffany, S.T. (1994). Comparisons of smoking urges elicited through imagery and *in vivo* cue exposure. Manuscript submitted for publication.

Drummond, D.C., Cooper, T. & Glautier, S.P. (1990). Conditioned learning in alcohol dependence: implications for cue exposure treatment. *British Journal of Addiction*, **85**, 725–743.

Elash, C.A., Tiffany, S.T. & Vrana, S.R. (1994). The manipulation of smoking urges through a brief imagery procedure: self-report, psychophysiological and startle-probe responses. *Experimental and Clinical Psychopharmacology*, in press.

Goldberg, S.R. & Schuster, C.R. (1970). Conditioned nalorphine-induced abstinence changes: persistence in post morphine-dependent monkeys. *Journal of the Experimental Analysis of Behavior*, **14**, 33–46.

Goudie, A.J. & Demellweek, C. (1986). Conditioning factors in drug tolerance.

In S.R. Goldberg & I.P. Stolerman (Eds) *Behavioral Analysis of Drug Dependence*, pp. 225–285. New York: Academic Press.

Gray, J.A. (1975). Elements of a Two-process Theory of Learning. London: Academic Press.

Greeley, J., Lê, D.A., Poulos, C.X. & Cappell, H. (1984). Alcohol is an effective cue in the conditional control of tolerance to alcohol. *Psychopharmacology*, **83**, 159–162.

Hinson, R.E., Poulos, C.X. & Cappell, H. (1982). Effects of pentobarbital and cocaine in rats expecting pentobarbitol. *Pharmacology, Biochemistry, and Behavior*, **16**, 661–666.

Holland, P.C. (1985). The nature of conditioned inhibition in serial and simultaneous feature negative discriminations. In R.R. Miller & N.E. Spear (Eds), *Information Processing in Animals: Conditioned Inhibition*, pp. 267–297. Hillsdale, NJ: Erlbaum.

Hull, J.G. & Bond, C.F. Jr (1986). Social and behavioral consequences of alcohol consumption: a meta-analysis. *Psychological Bulletin*, **99**, 347–360.

Hulse, S.H., Egeth, H. & Deese, J. (1980). *The Psychology of Learning*. New York: McGraw-Hill.

Jenkins, H.M. (1985). Conditioned inhibition of key pecking in the pigeon. In R.R. Miller & N.E. Spear (Eds), *Information Processing in Animals: Conditioned Inhibition*, pp. 327–353. Hillsdale, NJ: Erlbaum.

Johanson, C.E. (1990). Behavioral pharmacology, drug abuse, and the future. *Behavioural Pharmacology*, **1**, 385–393.

Kamin, L.J. & Brimer, C.J. (1963). The effects of intensity of conditioned and unconditioned stimuli on a conditioned emotional response. *Canadian Journal of Psychology*, **17**, 194–198.

Kamin, L.J., Brimer, C.J. & Black, A.H. (1963). Conditioned suppression as a monitor of fear of the CS in the course of avoidance training. *Journal of Comparative and Physiological Psychology*, **56**, 497–501.

King, D.A., Bouton, M.E. & Musty, R.E. (1987). Associative control of tolerance to the sedative effects of a short-acting benzodiazepine. *Behavioral Neuroscience*, **101**, 104–114.

Kruse, J.M., Overmier, J.B., Konz, W.A. & Rokke, E. (1983). Pavlovian conditioned stimulus effects upon instrumental choice behavior are reinforcer specific. *Learning and Motivation*, **14**, 165–181.

Levenson, R.W. (1992). Autonomic nervous system differences among emotions. *Psychological Science*, **3**, 23–27.

Levine, D.G. (1974). Needle freaks: compulsive self-injections by drug users. *American Journal of Psychiatry*, **131**, 297–300.

Levis, D.J. (1989). The case for a return to a two-factor theory of avoidance: the failure of non-fear interpretations. In S.B. Klein & R.R. Mowrer (Eds), *Contemporary Learning Theories*, pp. 227–277. Hillsdale, NJ: Lawrence Erlbaum.

Lubow, R.E. (1989). *Latent Inhibition and Conditioned Attention Theory*. Cambridge: Cambridge University Press.

Mackintosh, N.J. (1983). *Conditioning and Associative Learning*. New York: Oxford University Press.

Mackintosh, N.J. & Dickinson, A. (1979). Instrumental (Type II) conditioning. In A. Dickinson & R.A. Boakes (Eds), *Mechanisms of Learning and Motivation: A Memorial Volume to Jerzy Konorski*, pp. 143–169. Hillsdale, NJ: Erlbaum.

Markou, A., Weiss, F., Gold, L.H., Caine, S.B., Schulteis, G. & Koob, G.F. (1993). Animal models of drug craving. *Psychopharmacology*, **112**, 163–182.

Marlatt, G.A. & Gordon, J.R. (1980). Determinants of relapse: implications for the maintenance of behavior change. In P.O. Davidson & S.M. Davidson (Eds), *Behavioral Medicine: Changing Health Lifestyles*, pp. 410–452. New York: Brunner/Mazel.

Maude-Griffin, P.M. & Tiffany, S.T. (1989). Associative morphine tolerance in the rat: examinations of compensatory responding and cross-tolerance with stress-induced analgesia. *Behavioral and Neural Biology*, **51**, 11–33.

Maude-Griffin, P.M. & Tiffany, S.T. (1994). Verbal and physiological manifestations of smoking urges produced through imagery: role of affect and smoking abstinence. Manuscript submitted for publication.

McAuliffe, W.E., Feldman, B., Friedman, R., Lannes, E., Mahoney, C., Magnuson, E., Santangelo, S. & Ward, W. (1986). Explaining relapse to opiate addiction following completion of treatment. In F. Tims and C. Leukefeld (Eds), *Relapse and Recovery in Drug Abuse*, National Institute on Drug Abuse Research Monograph. Washington, DC: US Government Printing Office.

Mineka, S. (1979). The role of fear in theories of avoidance learning, flooding, and extinction. *Psychological Bulletin*, **86**, 985–1010.

Mineka, S. (1985). Animal models of anxiety-based disorders: their usefulness and limitations. In A.H. Tuma & J. Maser (Eds), *Anxiety and the Anxiety Disorders*, pp. 199–244. Hillsdale, NJ: Erlbaum.

Mowrer, O.H. (1947). On the dual nature of learning: a reinterpretation of "conditioning" and "problem-solving". *Harvard Educational Review*, **17**, 102–150.

Niaura, R.S., Rohsenow, D.J., Binkoff, J.A., Monti, P.M., Pedraza, M. & Abrams, D.B. (1988). Relevance of cue reactivity to understanding alcohol and smoking relapse. *Journal of Abnormal Psychology*, **97**, 133–152.

O'Brien, C.P. (1976). Experimental analysis of conditioning factors in human narcotic addiction. In L.S. Harris (Ed.), *Problems of Drug Dependence*, National Institute on Drug Abuse Research Monograph 27. Washington, DC: US Government Printing Office.

O'Brien, C.P., Chaddock, B., Woody, G. & Greenstein, R. (1974). Systematic extinction of addiction-associated rituals using narcotic antagonists. *Psychosomatic Medicine*, **36**, 458.

O'Brien, C.P., Greenstein, R., Ternes, J., McLellan, A.T. & Grabowski, J. (1980). Unreinforced self-injections: effects on rituals and outcome in heroin addicts. In L. Harris (Ed.), *Problems of Drug Dependence: Proceedings of the 41st Annual Scientific Meeting, The Committee on Problems of Drug Dependence, Inc.*, National Institute on Drug Abuse Research Monograph No. 27, pp. 275–281. Washington, DC: US Government Printing Office.

O'Brien, C.P., Childress, A.R., McLellan, A.T., Ehrman, R. & Ternes, J.W. (1988). Types of conditioning found in drug-dependent humans. In B.A. Ray (Ed.), *Learning Factors in Substance Abuse*, National Institute on Drug Abuse Research Monograph Series, pp. 44–61. Washington, DC: US Government Printing Office.

Obrist, P.A., Webb, R.A., Sutterer, J.R. & Howard, J.L. (1970). The cardia-somatic relationship: some reformulations; *Psychophysiology*, **6**, 569–587.

Peterson, G.B. & Trapold, M.A. (1980). Effects of altering outcome expectancies on pigeons' delayed conditional discrimination performance. *Learning and Motivation*, **11**, 267–288.

Poulos, C.X. & Cappell, H. (1991). Homeostatic theory of drug tolerance: a general model of physiological adaptation. *Psychological Review*, **98**, 390–408.

Poulos, C.X., Hinson, R. & Siegel, S. (1981). The role of Pavlovian processes in drug tolerance and dependence: implications for treatment. *Addictive Behaviors*, **6**, 205–211.

Rescorla, R.A. (1985). Conditioned inhibition and facilitation. In R.R. Miller & N.E. Spear (Eds), *Information Processing in Animals: Conditioned Inhibition*, pp. 299–326. Hillsdale, NJ: Lawrence Erlbaum.

Rescorla, R.A. (1988). Pavlovian conditioning: it's not what you think it is. *American Psychologist*, **43**, 151–160.

Rescorla, R.A. (1990). Evidence for an association between the discriminative stimulus and the response–outcome association in instrumental learning. *Journal of Experimental Psychology: Animal Behavior Processes*, **16**, 326–334.

Rescorla, R.A. (1991). Associative relations in instrumental learning: the Eighteenth Bartlett Memorial Lecture. *Quarterly Journal of Experimental Psychology*, **43B**, 1–23.

Rescorla, R.A. & Solomon, R.A. (1967). Two-process learning theory: relationships between Pavlovian conditioning and instrumental learning. *Psychological Review*, **74**, 151–182.

Robinson, T.E. & Berridge, K.C. (1993). The neural basis of drug craving: an incentive-sensitization theory of addiction, *Brain Research Reviews*, **18**, 247–291.

Rohsenow, D.J., Niaura, R.S., Childress, A.R., Abrams, D.B. & Monti, P.M. (1990). Cue reactivity in addictive behaviors: theoretical and treatment implications. *International Journal of the Addictions*, **25**, 957–993.

Ross, R.T. (1983). Relationships between the determinants of performance in serial feature-positive discriminations. *Journal of Experimental Psychology Animal Behavior Processes*, **9**, 349–373.

Schlosberg, H. (1937). The relationship between success and the laws of conditioning. *Psychological Review*, **44**, 379–394.

Schuster, C.R. & Thompson, T. (1961). Self-administration of and behavioral dependence on drugs. *Annual Review of Pharmacology*, **9**, 483–502.

Siegel, S. (1975). Evidence from rats that morphine tolerance is a learned response. *Journal of Comparative and Physiological Psychology*, **89**, 498–506.

Siegel, S. (1983). Classical conditioning, drug tolerance and drug dependence. In Y. Israel, F.B. Glaser, H. Kalant, R.E. Popham, W. Schmidt & R.G. Smart (Eds), *Research Advances in Alcohol and Drug Problems*, Vol. 7, pp. 207–246. New York: Plenum Press.

Siegel, S. (1989). Pharmacological conditioning and drug effects. In A.J. Goudie and M.W. Emmett-Oglesby (Eds), *Psychoactive Drugs: Tolerance and Sensitization*, pp. 115–180. Clifton, NJ: Humana Press.

Skinner, B.F. (1938). *The Behavior of Organisms*. New York: Appleton-Century.

Stephens, R. (1977). Psychophysiological variables in cigarette smoking and reinforcing effects of nicotine. *Addictive Behaviors*, **2**, 1–7.

Stewart, J., de Wit, H. & Eikelboom, R. (1984). Role of unconditioned and conditioned drug effects in self-administration of opiates and stimulants. *Psychological Review*, **91**, 251–268.

Tiffany, S.T. (1988). *Contemporary theories of drug urges, conflicting data, and an alternative cognitive framework*. Paper presented at the Conference on Theory and Research in Psychopathology, Performance, and Cognition, Gainsville, FL.

Tiffany, S.T. (1990). A cognitive model of drug urges and drug-use behavior: role of automatic and nonautomatic processes. *Psychological Review*, **97**, 147–168.

Tiffany, S.T. & Baker, T.B. (1981). Morphine tolerance in rats: congruence with Pavlovian paradigm. *Journal of Comparative and Physiological Psychology*, **95**, 747–762.

Tiffany, S.T. & Baker, T.B. (1986). Tolerance to alcohol: psychological models and their application to alcoholism. *Annals of Behavioral Medicine*, **8**, 7–12.

Tiffany, S.T. & Drobes, D.J. (1990). Imagery and smoking urges: the manipulation of affective content. *Addictive Behaviors*, **15**, 531–539.

Tiffany, S.T. & Hakenewerth, D.M. (1991). The production of smoking urges through an imagery manipulation: psychophysiological and verbal manifestations. *Addictive Behaviors*, **16**, 389–400.

Tiffany, S.T. & Maude-Griffin, P.M. (1988). Tolerance to morphine in the rat: associative and nonassociative effects. *Behavioral Neurosciences*, **102**, 534–543.

Tiffany, S.T. Cepeda-Benito, A. & Sanderson, L. (1994). Conditioned morphine tolerance: absence of compensatory responding across three tests of pain responding. Manuscript in preparation.

Tiffany, S.T., Drobes, D.J. & Cepeda-Benito, A. (1992). Contribution of associative and nonassociative processes to the development of morphine tolerance. *Psychopharmacology*, **109**, 185–190.

Tiffany, S.T., Maude-Griffin, P.M. & Drobes, D.J. (1991). The effect of inter-dose interval on the development of associative and nonassociative tolerance. *Behavioral Neuroscience*, **105**, 49–61.

Tiffany, S.T., Petrie, E.C., Baker, T.B. & Dahl, J. (1983). Conditioned morphine tolerance in the rat: absence of a compensatory response and cross-tolerance with stress. *Behavioral Neuroscience*, **97**, 335–353.

Weingarten, H.P. (1983). Conditioned cues elicit feeding in sated rats: a role for learning in meal initiation. *Science*, **220**, 431–432.

Wikler, A. (1948). Recent progress in research on the neurophysiological basis of morphine addiction. *American Journal of Psychiatry*, **105**, 329–338.

Wikler, A. (1972). Sources of reinforcement for drug using behavior—a theoretical formulation. In *Pharmacology and the Future of Man. Proceedings of 5th International Congress of Pharmacology*, Vol. 1, pp. 18–30. Basel: Karger.

Wikler, A. (1974). Requirements for extinction of relapse-facilitating variables and for rehabilitation in a narcotic-antagonist treatment program. *Advances in Biochemical Psychopharmacology*, Vol. 8, pp. 399–414 [Taken from M.C. Braude, L.S. Harris, E.L. May, J.P. Smith & J.E. Villarreal (Eds), *Narcotic Antagonists*. New York: Raven Press.]

Wikler, A. & Pescor, F.T. (1967). Classical conditioning of a morphine abstinence phenomenon, reinforcement of opioid-drinking behavior and "relapse" in morphine-addicted rats. *Psychopharmacologia*, **10**, 255–284.

Wise, R.A. (1988). The neurobiology of craving: implications for understanding and treatment of addiction. *Journal of Abnormal Psychology*, **97**, 118–132.

Young, A.M. & Herling, S. (1986). Drugs as reinforcers: studies in laboratory animals. In S.R. Goldberg & I.P. Stolerman (Eds), *Behavioral Analysis of Drug Dependence*, pp. 9–67. New York: Academic Press.

SECTION II   Methods of Studying Human Drug Cue Reactivity

CHAPTER 4   Methodological issues in cue reactivity research

Steven Glautier* and Stephen T. Tiffany[†]

INTRODUCTION

This chapter provides an overview of critical methodological issues in contemporary cue reactivity research. Three areas are covered. First, examples of designs employed in cue reactivity research are described and their limitations and advantages are discussed. Second, a number of different measures of cue reactivity have been used in previous research; these will be described and discussed with psychometric and heuristic considerations in mind. Finally, selected procedural issues in cue reactivity studies will be addressed. A tenet of the chapter is that the merits of decisions with regard to the three areas covered will have to be evaluated in terms of the explicit theoretical and/or clinical goals of the particular investigation. No single cue reactivity procedure can adequately resolve the myriad questions addiction researchers might wish to address. Certain combinations and qualities of procedures are better suited than others for investigating particular issues.

In order to illustrate the way in which some designs are better suited to answer particular theoretical and/or clinical questions, consider the following two experiments looking at the role of drug cues in the expression of tolerance to drug effects. It is now well established that both operant and Pavlovian processes play a part in drug tolerance (Young & Goudie, in press, Goldberg & Stolerman, 1986), and the two experiments to be described have Pavlovian processes as their foci. Although there are different models of the way in which Pavlovian conditioning works to produce the phenomenon of conditioned tolerance

*National Addiction Centre, University of London, UK, and [†]Purdue University, West Lafayette, Indiana, USA.

Addictive Behaviour: Cue Exposure Theory and Practice.
Edited by D.C. Drummond, S.T. Tiffany, S. Glautier and B. Remington.
© 1995 John Wiley & Sons Ltd.

(e.g. Baker & Tiffany, 1985; Siegel, 1989), all share two primary features, namely, each drug-taking episode is conceived of as a conditioning trial in which the stimuli present during drug taking acquire conditioned stimulus (CS) properties signalling the impending arrival of a powerful drug effect or unconditioned stimulus (US); and the presence of established CSs for drug administration results in a smaller apparent UR effect. Of course, this means that a drug given in the absence of the usual CSs (i.e. unexpectedly) will have a larger effect.

Ehrman et al. (1992) conducted a study in which six detoxified opiate addicts were given doses of hydromorphone under two different administration conditions. One hydromorphone dose was self-administered by the addicts following a cook-up ritual while the other dose was given by infusion. The responses elicited by these two conditions were compared with responses produced by an infusion of saline. In keeping with the predictions of models of conditioned tolerance, the heart rate and skin temperature effects of hydromorphone were larger for a subgroup of subjects when it was given by infusions (i.e. in the absence of drug CSs). Furthermore, responses elicited by self-administration of hydromorphone did not differ from those produced in the saline infusion condition. This experiment provides some support for the arguments put forward by Siegel (1984, 1989) to account for instances of heroin overdose. Overdoses may occur even when the dose administered is the same as that which has previously been well tolerated. This often happens when the circumstances of drug administration change, presumably because the changed circumstances result in the absence of the usual drug CSs. Thus, one of the strengths of the Ehrman et al. experiment was its evaluation of a clinically important phenomenon in the clinical population for whom it is of most relevance. However, one shortcoming of the study is that the design precluded any convincing demonstration that the observed effects were due to conditioning or even represented opioid tolerance. Although the face validity of this type of study is high, unless conditioning is actually carried out by the experimenter, the results must be interpreted cautiously.

The second experiment, carried out by Dafters & Anderson (1982), was unable to provide a clear demonstration of such a clinically relevant effect but, nevertheless, was able to provide a more compelling demonstration of the role of classical conditioning in the production of tolerance. Dafters & Anderson used a healthy group of volunteer subjects, each of whom attended the laboratory for 14 experimental sessions. During the sessions, subjects consumed either alcoholic or soft drinks in one of two different distinctive rooms. The consumption of the drinks was arranged such that one of the experimental rooms was always associated with alcohol consumption whereas the other room was always paired with soft drinks. In this way it was predicted that the alcohol- and soft drink-paired distinctive rooms would acquire different conditioned properties. Over the course of the sessions, it was found that the heart rate effects of alcohol diminished, indicating the development of tolerance. On a test session in which alcohol was given in the soft drink room (i.e. unexpectedly), tolerance to alcohol's heart rate effects was lost, but it was reinstated on a subsequent test in which alcohol was again administered in its usual CS context.

In summary, it seems that certain experimental designs may be better suited than others to address particular questions. Ethical and practical considerations limit the kinds of studies that can be carried out with both addict and non-addict subjects. Nevertheless, it is possible to obtain evidence for conditioning effects in other experimental designs and, as with the Ehrman et al. (1992) study, collect more clinically relevant data in an opportunistic experiment (see below). Were these the only two experiments to demonstrate these effects, one would have to remain sceptical about the whole concept of conditioned tolerance and its clinical implications. However, the convergence of data from a variety of sources, including the strong evidence of conditioned tolerance effects from animal investigations (e.g. Cepeda-Benito & Tiffany, 1992; Tiffany, Maude-Griffin & Drobes, 1991; Tiffany, Drobes & Cepeda-Benito, 1992), provides convincing support for the contention that classical conditioning can contribute to the development of drug tolerance.

EXPERIMENTAL DESIGN IN CUE REACTIVITY STUDIES

As will be discussed below, studies of cue reactivity have been carried out with a variety of dependent measures and procedures. However, central to every study is the attempt to identify (a) differences in responses elicited by drug-related and neutral stimuli, and/or (b) differences in responses elicited by drug-related stimuli amongst different groups of subjects. A core assumption of cue reactivity investigations is that stimuli previously associated with drug taking will elicit distinctive patterns of responses because of the drug user's history of experiences with those stimuli. However, the majority of cue reactivity studies are not adequate to make a direct test of the impact of drug history on reactivity as the different histories are usually assumed, rather than produced experimentally. Studies in which the histories are assumed can be termed opportunistic investigations; those in which associations between drug and other stimuli are manipulated by the researcher can be termed conditioning experiments.

Opportunistic Investigations

Opportunistic cue reactivity studies are those in which the investigators look for evidence that drug cues have characteristic response-eliciting capacities, but their defining feature is that they rely on their subjects' extra-experimental drug-use histories. Thus, if one was interested in how physiological responses to the sight of a cigarette were altered by a conditioning history in which cigarette cues had previously been associated with a bolus of nicotine, one might present smokers and non-smokers with cigarettes. If smokers responded with a larger heart rate increase than the non-smokers, it might be concluded that previous conditioning contributed to this observation. Such a finding would indeed be compatible with that conclusion, but there may be many other factors at work. For instance, smokers might respond differently to any stimulus or non-smokers could orient more strongly to the relatively novel stimulus provided by the cigarette; heart rate decelerations often occur during attention to environmental stimuli (Lacey, 1967). Such variables might be accommodated by treating them as "nuisance" parameters (Everitt & Dunn, 1991) whose effects might be statistically isolated from the effects of conditioning history. This could be achieved by measuring general responsivity to stimuli and including it as a term in a statistical analysis. Unfortunately, a statistical solution to the problem of pre-existing group differences on a nuisance variable is rarely justified either logically or statistically (e.g. Meehl, 1971; Woodward & Goldstein, 1977). Alternatively, one could attempt to match the relative familiarity of the control and experimental stimuli. However, a simple matching strategy may only address the potential impact of one confounding stimulus dimension; there may be many other differences across stimuli other than conditioning history accounting for variations in reactivity. Moreover, matching on one dimension may systematically unmatch stimuli on other critical dimensions.

Fortunately, there are alternative designs that can be used in opportunistic experiments on cue reactivity. These designs carry their own difficulties but do address some of the inadequacies inherent in procedures that simply compare groups with different drug-use histories. First among these is the design in which within-subject comparisons are made between stimuli assumed to have different conditioning histories. In a recent study by Glautier & Drummond (1994), alcoholic patients going through a cue exposure treatment (Drummond & Glautier, 1994) were presented with two different kinds of beverage, a favourite alcoholic and a favourite soft drink, before their treatments began. It was found that skin conductance and self-reported tension and desire to drink were all higher in the presence of the alcoholic drink. Although several weaknesses associated with a between-group comparison are circumvented in such a design, it is still possible that differences between the alcoholic and soft drink other than drug-use history are responsible for the patterns of effects. For example, disparities in familiarity or sensory intensity of the stimuli may account for response differences. McCaul, Turkkan & Stitzer (1989b) attempted to take the intensity factor into account in a study in which subjects exposed to whiskey, water, and pepper juice. The taste of whiskey and pepper juice were both rated as more intense than the water and they both elicited greater heart rate and skin conductance responses.

Newlin et al. (1989) took this approach further by employing four different stimuli that subjects had to smell; each stimulus was intended to control one particular factor that might have been confounded with drug-use history. Subjects were presented with water, a favourite non-alcoholic drink, a favourite alcoholic drink, and a sweet roll. In his way one could hope to partial out the effect of smelling itself (water control), the effect of smelling a desirable beverage (non-alcoholic drink), and the effect of smelling something with a food value (sweet roll). An additional feature of Newlin et al.'s study was the comparison of reactivity across these stimuli in groups of alcoholic and non-alcoholic subjects. Therefore, this design allowed for a comparison of reactivity profiles across subject groups and stimulus types. The objective was to triangulate the effects of drug-use history by having some controls for between-subject and between-stimulus differences.

In summary, three basic opportunistic study designs can be identified. First, comparisons can be made between the responses to drug-related stimuli in different subject groups assumed to vary systematically in conditioning histories. Second, drug-related cues and neutral control stimuli can be presented to subjects with a history of drug use. Each of these alternatives present interpretational problems. Between-stimulus comparisons may confound many irrelevant differences between test stimuli with any differences in conditioning history. Between-subject comparisons risk confounding any differences in the conditioning history of addict populations and control subjects with other group differences. A third "mixed" design uses addicts and non-addicts presented with drug-related and neutral stimuli in the hope that differences between subject populations will be the same for different stimuli and that unconditioned differences between stimuli will be the same across subject groups; differences between drug and neutral cues attributable to conditioning history are suggested if the drug-neutral difference is different in the addict population. However, this merely pushes the basic problem a step further away. One is bound to ask, what if subject and stimulus factors interact in some way to produce response differences that are still not due to conditioning? In responding to stimuli in general, what if alcoholics simply show a greater increase in reaction per unit increase in stimulus intensity than do non-alcoholic controls? For example, if the sight of an alcoholic drink unconditionally elicits larger responses than the sight of orange juice then if the alcohol-neutral difference is greater in alcoholics we may inadvertently conclude this difference is due to their conditioning history.

Robbins & Ehrman (1992) suggested that some of the limitations of opportunistic designs might be overcome by using arousal control and crossover response designs. Arousal control assumes that drug stimuli are somehow more arousing in general than are typical control stimuli. Therefore, they recommend using non-drug control stimuli that are themselves arousing. The value of such an approach is doubtful for several reasons. First, it rests on the untested presumption that arousal is more important to control than other dimensions such as familiarity or intensity. Moreover, the behavioural and physiological manifestations of arousal are clearly heterogeneous, making it nearly impossible to comprehensively match arousal profiles across drug and non-drug stimuli. Finally, the logic of "arousal control" assumes that any arousing properties of drug-relevant stimuli develop independently of an addict's drug use. In fact, drug stimuli may be more arousing precisely because of the addict's conditioning history. The crossover response design involves two groups of addicts, for example, one of which uses heroin and the other of which uses cocaine. These subjects are then presented with cues appropriate for heroin and cocaine use. Cocaine addicts should respond selectively to the cocaine cues whereas the reverse should be true for the heroin addicts. Unfortunately, using another group of addicts as controls may be no better than using non-addicts unless it can be shown that the two addict groups are more similar on one or more relevant nuisance parameters than are addict and non-addict subjects. Therefore, this design simply boils down to an elaboration on the basic approach using a mixture of different subject groups and different stimuli.

Conditioning Experiments

Robbins & Ehrman (1992) argued that the only way to establish that different responding to drug and neutral cues is due to classical conditioning is for the experimenter actually to do the conditioning rather than to rely upon opportunistic designs. Although opportunistic studies have considerable practical merit, we agree that only conditioning experiments, with the appropriate controls, can establish that a response to a drug-relevant stimulus represents the operation of classical conditioning (see also Tiffany, 1992). The objective of a conditioning study is to examine whether or not different responses to cues for a drug develop as a result of a history in which the cues act as signals for drug delivery. In order to do this, the principal independent variable is the contingency or relationship between the drug cue and delivery of the drug. Figure 4.1 illustrates different degrees of contingency between CSs and USs.

In the top line, (P(US|CS) = 100%), the occurrence of the CS predicts the US perfectly; every time the CS occurs the US follows. In the lines below, P(US|CS) is degraded by scheduling CSs at times othat than when the US is imminent. In the final case (P(US|CS) = 0%), the CS is actually predictive of the absence of the US. A CS that predicts the absence of an otherwise expected US is usually termed an inhibitory CS, or CS−, whereas a CS predicting the US is termed an excitatory CS, or CS+. In the case of the middle line, where P(US|CS) = 50%, the CS is neutral and may be termed CS0. The recognition of this gradient from excitatory to inhibitory conditioning has been fundamental to current understanding of conditioning processes. Its significance can be understood if the 50%

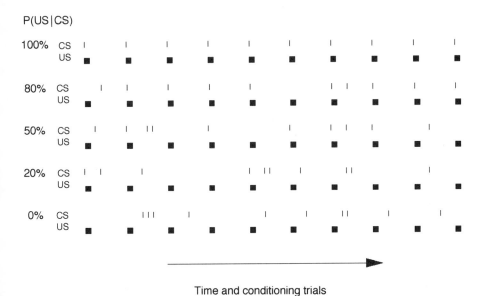

Time and conditioning trials

Figure 4.1 An illustration of different CS–US arrangements showing different degrees of contingency between CS and US. In the top line the CS is always followed by the US, in the bottom line the US never follows the CS. Intermediate degrees of contingency are shown in the three middle lines.

group in the figure is contrasted with a group for which there had been equal numbers of CS–US pairings but for whom neither the CS nor the US occurred at other times. It would be expected that the latter group would show more conditioning than the 50% group. In fact, even if P(US|CS) = 40%, good conditioning can be produced, and interpolating additional USs between CS–US pairings so that P(US|no CS) = 40% abolishes that conditioning (Rescorla, 1968).

There are a large number of different kinds of design for classical conditioning experiments, so much so that Turkkan (1989, p. 122) has used the term "a candy store approach" to describe the way in which investigators have adopted different controls. We shall consider two basic designs, the differential conditioning procedure and the truly random control procedure. In both designs, it is possible to ensure that comparisons are not made between groups of subjects that have had different degrees of CS or US exposure therefore minimizing the risk that changes in response to CSs are due to sensitization or pseudoconditioning (Harris, 1943; Wickens & Wickens, 1942). As an example of the problems for designs in which comparisons are made between groups with different amounts of US exposure, consider the experiment by McCaul, Turkkan & Stitzer (1989a). Half of their subjects received an orange-flavoured drink containing alcohol on four occasions while the other half received a non-alcoholic orange drink on four occasions. On the fifth occasion, all subjects received the non-alcoholic orange drink and contrasts between the responses to the consumption of these drinks were made between groups, apparently showing good conditioning effects on heart rate and skin conductance. Unfortunately, the degree of US exposure and level of CS–US contingency were confounded in this study. Consequently, the experimental group may have had a different response on the test session than the control group because they had more US exposures. The experimental group may have also responded differently from the controls because they may have noticed that the flavour of the drink changed from the conditioning to the test session.

The differential conditioning procedure is a within-subject design; each subject experiences two CSs, one of which is established as CS+ whereas the other is established as CS–, corresponding to contingency arrangements in the top (100%) and bottom (0%) lines of Figure 4.1. This arrangement is a special case of an explicitly unpaired procedure and has, since the origins of research into classical conditioning, frequently been found to produce a rapid and reliable differentiation of responses to the two CSs (Pavlov, 1927). A design in which drug delivery is explicitly paired or unpaired with distinctive environmental cues has become the standard for animal research on conditioned tolerance effects (e.g. Cepeda-

Benito & Tiffany, 1992; Tiffany, Maude-Griffin & Drobes, 1991; Tiffany, Drobes & Cepeda-Benito, 1992). A differential design was used in the experiment carried out by Glautier, Drummond & Remington (1994), which is described in more detail by Glautier & Remington (Chapter 2). In this type of differential design, in order to rule out the possibility that the unconditioned properties of the CSs used do not result in apparent conditioning effect, it is necessary to do one of two things. Either it must be shown that the two CSs do not result, prior to conditioning, in different responses, or that the CS functions of the two CSs must be counterbalanced across two subgroups of subjects.

An essential issue for the differential design is the potential inhibitory impact of the CS– on the test response (Pavlov, 1927; Rescorla, 1967). This presents no difficulties at all if the responses to CS+ and CS– have opposing valences or if the response to CS– is simply behaviourally silent until it is measured indirectly (e.g. by its effects on responding to CS+s (summation test) or by the subsequent difficulty transforming the CS– into a CS+ (retardation test)). An example in which CS+ and CS– had opposing valence was described by Rescorla (1966). He presented CS+, CS– and CS0 to three groups of dogs working on a Sidman shock avoidance schedule. The CS+ dogs had previously experienced shocks after the CS, the CS– dogs in contrast had the absence of shock signalled by the CS, whereas the CS0 dogs experienced the CS and US in random relations. Presentation of CS+ resulted in an increase in the avoidance rate, CS– resulted in a decreased rate, and CS0 resulted in no change. However, if CS+ and CS– result in the same kind of response, for example, both produce an increase in skin conductance, then comparing CS+ and CS– may result in a failure to detect experimental effects. Unfortunately while modern approaches to Pavlovian learning (e.g. Wagner & Brandon, 1989; Hall, 1991) offer a sophisticated account of associative processes, the translation of this learning into performance is difficult to predict (cf. Glautier and Remington, Chapter 2) so neither the divergence of responses to CS+ and CS– nor the behavioural silence of CS– is likely to be universal across all response systems and conditioning paradigms.

One solution to this problem is to adopt, as Rescorla (1966) did, a truly random (CS0) control. Several implementations of this procedure are possible but one incorporates a between-subjects factor; for the experimental group CS+ and CS– are established in the same way as for the differential design, but for the control group both CSs are experienced so that they neither predict the US nor its absence. Table 4.1 illustrates this design and contrasts it with the differential design previously described. Both designs are optimal in the sense that both CSs used are experienced an equal number of times (within and between groups) and

Table 4.1 Illustration of a basic differential conditioning design and one with a truly random control group

Differential design	Truly random control design Group 1	Group 2
CS1 → Alcohol	CS1 → Alcohol	CS1 → Alcohol
CS2 → Soft	CS2 → Soft	CS2 → Soft
CS1 → Alcohol	CS1 → Alcohol	CS1 → Soft
CS2 → Soft	CS2 → Soft	CS2 → Alcohol
CS1 → Alcohol	CS1 → Alcohol	CS1 → Alcohol
CS2 → Soft	CS2 → Soft	CS2 → Soft
CS1 → Alcohol	CS1 → Alcohol	CS1 → Soft
CS2 → Soft	CS2 → Soft	CS2 → Alcohol

NB In practice there would be additional cells in order to incorporate counterbalancing of CS+ and CS– functions across CS1 and CS2, and to deal with order effects.

the US (alcohol) is experienced the same number of times as is its absence (soft drink), again both within and between groups. In this design, comparisons can be made between CS+ and CS– within the experimental group and contrasts can also be made between groups. A serious limitation of the truly random control design is the extra subject requirement and the fact that the control group's responding may not stabilize for many trials.

MEASUREMENT OF CUE REACTIVITY

Cue reactivity can be measured in three domains of human functioning, namely, self-report, physiological responses, and overt actions. These will be considered in turn.

Self-report Measures

A variety of self-report measures have been collected in cue reactivity studies including assessments of drug craving, drug withdrawal, mood, drug outcome expectancies, self-efficacy, and attributions. Of all the self-report measures, craving or urge report is collected most frequently. Despite the putative theoretical and clinical importance of craving, nearly all researchers utilize single-item questionnaires of unknown reliability or validity when assessing this construct. Tiffany (1992) has noted that the reliability and sensitivity of single-item craving questionnaires are likely to be low. Furthermore, single-item questionnaires cannot capture possible multidimensional features of craving report. A recent series of craving questionnaires developed by Tiffany and his colleagues provide a more complete evaluation of self-reported craving for cigarettes (Tiffany & Drobes, 1991), cocaine (Tiffany et al., 1993), heroin (Tiffany et al., 1994), and alcohol (Singleton, Tiffany & Henningfield, 1994). These instruments, which range in length from 32 to 45 items, may be too long to use as primary dependent measures in many cue reactivity studies. However, brief forms of these questionnaires have been developed and, in the case of urges for cigarettes, systematically employed in several cue reactivity investigations (e.g. Burton & Tiffany, 1994; Cepeda-Benito & Tiffany, 1994; Elash, Tiffany & Vrana, 1995; Drobes & Tiffany, 1994).

Mood or affective state has also been assessed frequently as a self-report manifestation of cue reactivity. As with craving, most mood measures used in this research consist of single-item questionnaires which have not been validated. Some investigators have created brief multi-item mood scales using items selected, in some cases, from longer questionnaires of mood states (e.g. Payne et al., 1991; Sherman et al., 1989; Powell, Bradley & Gray, 1992). These homemade, multi-item mood questionnaires are used typically with no evaluation of their psychometric properties, and it is possible that their reliability is considerably less than generally assumed (Watson, Clark & Tellegen, 1988). However, there are several comprehensive, psychometrically sound instruments for the assessment of specific mood states and general levels of positive and negative affect. As one example, a nine-item questionnaire developed by Diener & Emmons (1984) provides a reliable and sensitive evaluation of intensity of positive and negative mood that can be incorporated readily into cue reactivity investigations (e.g. Maude-Griffin & Tiffany, 1994; Burton, Drobes & Tiffany, 1992).

The psychometric weaknesses of cue reactivity studies are not limited to craving or mood measures. Cue reactivity researchers rarely attend to the psychometric adequacy of their self-report, physiological or behavioural measures. In general, an unreliable, insensitive measure of any sort cannot accurately reflect the impact of cue manipulations, reveal the true magnitude of relationships between one measure and another, or provide a meaningful evaluation of the relative influence of cue manipulations on one variable versus another. More comprehensive and reliable assessments of self-reported craving and mood states are now available, but the theoretical and clinical utility of the entire cue reactivity research endeavour will be limited without greater attention to basic psychometric considerations across all domains of reactivity.

Physiological Measures

There is a multitude of physiological measures that might be assessed in a cue reactivity study, and a consideration of the promise and problems associated with specific measures is well beyond the scope of this chapter. Although advances in hardware and software have made it easier and less costly for cue reactivity researchers to gather an increasing diversity of physiological data, these technical innovations have in no way diminished the formidable methodological and conceptual issues confronting the measurement and interpretation of psychophysiological measures. Therefore, the cue reactivity researcher wishing to evaluate physiological variables must be attuned to technological, methodological, psychometric, and theoretical issues relevant to general psychophysiological investigations (e.g. Cacioppo & Tassinary, 1990a; Coles, Porges & Donchin, 1986).

The full potential of psychophysiological assessment in cue reactivity research has been limited by two factors. First, the selection of physiological measures in many studies often appears to be guided more by convenience or what's available on the researcher's polygraph than by theoretically or clinically motivated decisions. For example, Tiffany (1992) noted that, although animal conditioning research with alcohol has consistently identified only one response that might be indicative of a classically conditioned response to stimuli paired with alcohol delivery (core hyperthermia; see review by Goudie & Demellweek, 1986), this response has not been systematically evaluated in cue reactivity research with alcoholics. As another example, there is a considerable literature on the role of classical conditioning in tolerance to the analgesic effects of morphine (Baker & Tiffany, 1985; Siegel, 1983; Young & Goudie, 1994), yet there is a paucity of research on the impact of drug cues on nociceptive responding in opiate addicts.

The second problem confronting psychophysiological assessment in cue reactivity research is the tendency of many investigators to portray any physiological reaction to drug-relevant stimuli as necessarily and solely indicative of a classically conditioned response. This interpretation, which assumes a one-to-one relationship between a psychological process (conditioning) and a physiological reaction, can rarely be justified in psychophysiological research (Cacioppo & Tassinary, 1990b) unless, as discussed earlier, carefully designed experiments are carried out. It is likely that any given response to a drug stimulus reflects a variety of psychologically relevant processes, only one of which might be conditioning (see Tiffany, Chapter 3). Moreover, an exclusive focus on conditioning interpretations diverts attention from the role of other psychological processes that may mediate reactions to drug-related stimuli, processes that may have important implications for understanding and treating addictive behaviour. For example, Tiffany (1990) has hypothesized that many cue reactions represent the immediate cognitive and behavioural demands of the stimulus situation. This conceptualization suggests that physiological reactions may yield fruitful indicators of cognitive processes evoked by the presentation of drug cues to addicts. Although it may be important to evaluate the specific role of conditioning processes in cue reactivity, cue reactivity may be important in addiction even if its immediate origins lie in other psychological processes.

The most commonly collected physiological variables in studies of cue reactivity represent measures of autonomic functioning such as heart rate, blood pressure, skin conductance, and salivation. The implicit and reasonable assumption in these studies is that cue-specific changes in autonomic measures are indirect indices of central nervous system activity. With few exceptions (e.g. Ludwig, Wikler & Stark, 1974), more direct measures of brain activity have not been utilized in cue reactivity research. Recent advances in a variety of brain imaging techniques (e.g. quantitative EEG, magnetoencephalography, cerebral blood flow) permit the evaluation of more direct indices of brain functioning as additional measures of cue reactivity (see Zappulla et al., 1991, for examples of applications of these technologies). At present, these measures are technologically demanding, expensive, and available to only a few researchers. If these measures of brain functioning are to advance our understanding of cue reactivity phenomena, they will have to be employed in cue reactivity paradigms having a clear record of producing robust effects with psychometrically sound measures and methodologically appropriate manipulations of drug cues. Equally important, unless the applications of these techniques are guided by explicit and fully articulated theoretical considerations regarding the nature of cue reactivity, the yield from these studies may not justify their expense.

Drug-use Measures

Relatively few studies have examined the impact of manipulations of drug cues on drug-use behaviour even though this is obviously the most important practical concern. When these behaviours have been assessed, it has almost always been the case that a single behaviour has been targeted, although the specific behaviours used to index drug use have varied considerably across studies. Some examples include number of lever presses for an alcoholic beverage (Ludwig, Wikler & Stark, 1974), speed of drinking (Hodgson, Rankin & Stockwell, 1979; Rankin, Hodgson & Stockwell, 1979), choice of alcoholic versus non-alcoholic beverage (Kaplan, Meyer & Stroebel, 1983), time spent smoking a cigarette (Rickard-Figueroa & Zeichner, 1985), and time spent completing a simple tracing task prior to gaining access to a cigarette (Wetter, Brandon & Baker, 1992).

Drug-use behaviours in addicts are extraordinarily complex, comprising a wide range of highly practised, specific actions integrated into co-ordinated sequences culminating in the ingestion of drug into the body. The selection of any one of these actions as necessarily representative of all the component actions is not likely to do justice to the multifaceted nature of drug-acquisition and drug-use sequences. At a general level, a distinction might be drawn between actions involved in securing drugs and those actions necessary to consume drugs. This distinction parallels the one made by some motivational and learning theorists between approach and consummatory behaviours (e.g. Bindra, 1974; Holman, 1975; Toates, 1986). Drug-use measures can also be divided into behaviours that reflect the naturally occurring drug-acquisition and drug-use repertoire of the addict (e.g. buying cocaine from a dealer, injecting heroin, smoking a cigarette), and more artificial laboratory-induced behaviours. These would be actions not represented in the natural drug-use behaviours of the addict but required in laboratory settings to gain access to drugs or to consume drugs. As an example of a laboratory-induced drug-acquisition behaviour, Ludwig, Wikler & Stark (1974) examined the impact of alcohol consumption and exposure to alcohol-related cues on the amount of lever pressing the subjects engaged in to obtain an alcohol reward. The two divisions suggested above yield four distinct categories of drug-use behaviour with representative examples as shown in Figure 4.2.

It is likely that the behaviours in each of these categories are influenced by a different mix of motivational, situational, and cognitive factors. These considerations have important implications for evaluating relationships between various indices of drug use and other measures of cue reactivity. For example, Tiffany (1990) predicted that self-reported craving will display weaker associations with measures of drug use that reflect highly practised or automatized behaviours than behaviours that are less extensively automatized. Using the categorizations outlined above, this theory would predict that measures of artificial acquisition and drug-use behaviours, which would be presumably less practised, would be more strongly correlated with self-reported craving than naturally occurring behaviours. Irrespective of the validity of these predictions, the categorization described above suggests the conventional,

	Acquisition approach	Consumption
Natural	Locating a drug pusher	Injecting heroin
Artificial	Lever presses for alcohol	Puffing from a cigarette-smoking device

Figure 4.2 Classification scheme for categorizing measures of drug-use behaviour with representative examples.

widespread depiction of drug-use behaviour as a unidimensional phenomenon that can be evaluated through any one of its components is inadequate.

Multi-domain Assessment

Although a focused study of cue reactivity in any one of the three domains described above is an entirely legitimate activity, most cue reactivity researchers collect measures from two or even all three domains in any given study. One assumption implicit in the conduct and interpretation of many of these studies is that measures from all domains index a unidimensional cue reactivity process. For example, it might be presumed that all measures reflect classical conditioning or that all measures arise from activation of a central craving state. This assumption is questionable, as, even within any one domain, there is little evidence of a unidimensional process controlling all responding (Tiffany, 1990). More generally, there is, as of yet, no clearly established way of predicting relationships between measures either within or across domains.

It is possible that multivariate techniques (e.g. Nesselroade & Cattell, 1988) could be used to help integrate and interpret these diverse data, but the value of such an approach will depend on two factors. First, it will require the development of psychometrically sound assessments of key variables within each domain. Second, the selection and interpretation of meaningful variables will depend upon the articulation of comprehensive theories of cue reactivity that accommodate and predict the diversity of reactions and interrelationships among measures that might be evoked by presentations of drug-relevant stimuli. Multivariate analyses on unreliable or insensitive measures, using data selection and analytic strategies not explicitly guided by theory, are unlikely to yield new insights into the critical psychological or biological mechanisms controlling cue reactions.

CUE REACTIVITY MANIPULATIONS

A diversity of procedures utilizing a variety of cues and settings have been employed in cue reactivity research. We will provide a brief account of some of the factors we regard as important in evaluating cue reactivity manipulations. These considerations have a bearing on the integration of the diverse results across studies and give a broad perspective on the kinds of investigations that could come under the general heading of cue reactivity research.

A basic issue in the design of any cue reactivity study will be what cue or cues should be presented (Laberg, 1990). A distinction might be drawn between external and internal cues; the first category consists of exteroceptive stimuli such as a drug-paired context, the sight and smell of a glass of beer, or the sight of somebody lighting a cigarette; the second consists of interoceptive states such as a mood, the stimulation produced by the initial effects of a drug, or drug withdrawal reactions.[1]

Perhaps due to the ease with which external cues can be manipulated, there are numerous examples of these kinds of procedures. For example, Pomerleau et al. (1983) had alcoholic and non-alcoholic subjects hold and smell either their favourite alcoholic drinks or cedar chips. In an experiment with opiate addicts, Powell et al. (1990) used either simulated drug-taking paraphernalia, or slides of other people using opiates. One important dimension upon which presentation of slide and "real" drug cues might differ is drug expectancy. In the case of slide presentation alone, drug expectancy may well be lower than when real drug cues are present. Given the importance of expectancy effects in producing differences in the observed effects of drugs (e.g. Marlatt & Rohsenow, 1980), it would seem important to study, or at least to control, the possibility that the expectancy of receiving a drug plays a part in producing responses to cues. It would therefore be instructive to compare responses to cook-up rituals, such as those used by Ehrman et al. (1992), in which subjects' expectancy of consuming drug was varied.

At the interface between the exteroceptive and interoceptive cue category is the class of experiments in which placebo versions of drugs are given.

The objective here is to ensure that subjects experience the full range of cues associated with consuming a drug without actually allowing the drug to enter the body. For example, Newlin (1985) gave subjects either a glass of Near Beer (a non-alcoholic beer) or a glass of 7 Up. Again, the problem area of drug expectancy crops up; the subjects in these two conditions would differ in their expectancies of drug effects, especially since the Near Beer subjects were told that their drinks were alcoholic. One solution to this problem would be to employ a variation on the balanced placebo design experiment in which cue (e.g. Near Beer versus 7 Up) was crossed with alcohol expectancy (e.g. told alcohol versus told soft). However, an apparently insoluble problem with placebo administration is that subjects may detect deception. At best, this may weaken experimental effects; at worst, results may be misleading. An indirect method of studying the effects of cues associated with the consumption of drinks, avoiding the problem of placebo administration, is the administration of drug plus or minus the usual accompanying cues. This strategy has been a mainstay of research into the role of cues in drug tolerance and an example of this design was described in the introduction (Dafters & Anderson, 1982).

Both mood states and drug effects have been considered to be particularly important kinds of internal cue. Surveys of relapse episodes in addicts have indicated the importance of moods, especially negative moods, as precursors of relapse (e.g. Marlatt & Gordon, 1980; Litman et al., 1983). A number of cue reactivity studies have been carried out in which mood has been manipulated through imagery (Burton, Drobes & Tiffany, 1992; Elash, Tiffany & Vrana, 1995; Maude-Griffin & Tiffany, 1994; Tiffany & Drobes, 1990), or hypnosis (Childress et al., 1987; Litt et al., 1990). These studies have found consistently that induction of negative mood can be a potent elicitor of drug craving. The effects of these manipulations on mood states have been evaluated through comprehensive measures of self-reported affect (e.g. Maude-Griffin & Tiffany, 1994) as well as with indices of facial electromyographic activity indicative of affective processing (e.g. Burton, Drobes & Tiffany, 1992; Elash, Tiffany & Vrana, 1995).

Drug effects, especially priming doses of the drug of addiction (e.g. alcohol for the abstinent alcoholic), have attracted attention particularly in the light of Jellinek's (1952) writings on loss of control. Establishing the impact of drug manipulations may seem more straightforward than evaluating the validity of mood manipulations, but given that there may be wide variations in the effects of drugs between individuals, and even within individuals on different occasions, this confidence may be misplaced. Wherever there is any doubt regarding a drug effect (e.g. in low dose conditions), it would seem necessary explicitly to assess the drug effect. If it is necessary to obtain a very precise effect, the dose can be titrated across subjects such that each individual has a functionally equivalent dose (Naitoh, 1972). Two kinds of drug cue effect have been studied; the first concerns the case in which a priming dose of a drug is given. Both Hodgson, Rankin & Stockwell (1979) and Stockwell et al. (1982) showed that priming doses of alcohol could increase the speed with which a subsequent alcoholic drink was consumed in alcoholic subjects. More recently, de Wit and Chutaupe (1993) used a choice procedure and found priming effects in social drinkers. Alcoholic drinks were chosen more often when subjects had been given priming drinks containing alcohol. The second kind of drug cue effect involves the investigation of administration of one drug on reactivity to other drug stimuli. For example, Nil, Buzzi & Battig (1984) and Mintz et al. (1985) found that doses of alcohol increased smoking as indexed by increases in puff volume, rate of smoking, and change in expired carbon monoxide levels. More recently, Burton & Tiffany (1994) demonstrated that alcohol intoxication increased craving to smoke in regular cigarette smokers but did not selectively enhance cue reactivity to actual or imaginal presentations of smoking-related stimuli.

CONCLUDING COMMENTS

The domain of cue reactivity research is of such size and scope that any realization of the opportunities it affords for understanding or treating addictive disorders requires mastery of a number of critical methodological, psychometric, and conceptual factors. In this chapter we have tried to address those issues with the greatest general relevance to cue reactivity work. These included basic considerations of experimental design as well as the selection, measurement and interpretation of dependent and independent measures, and an overview of some of the main paradigms which can be employed. We believe that systematic attention to these issues in the development, implementation, and analysis of cue reactivity investigations will yield many benefits. Not least among these is the prospect of developing a better understanding of the factors that contribute to the phenomenon of cue reactivity *per se*, and the possibility that a better understanding of cue reactivity may lead to the development of effective cue exposure treatments. It is important to point out that the investigation of cue reactivity and cue exposure treatments could go ahead independently; they are both substantial and interesting topics in their own right. However, because of the obvious links it will be of benefit for both fields to be closely allied.

NOTE

1. The categorization of external and internal cues is offered here as a means to loosely classify cue manipulations and is not meant to represent a fundamental partition of drug-relevant cues. On the one hand, all cues might be thought of as external in origin. For example, the initiation of a drug state requires the administration of a drug and the induction of a mood requires the presentation of affective material. On the other hand, all cues could be viewed as essentially internal, in the sense that they produce patterns of reactivity presumably through the mediation of some psychological processes. It could be argued, for instance, that a smoker watching someone smoke reacts to that situation only to the extent that those stimuli activate memory systems, and it is those internal states that provide the proximal cause for patterns of reactivity.

REFERENCES

Baker, T.B. & Tiffany, S.T. (1985). Morphine tolerance as habituation. *Psychological Review*, **92**, 78–108.

Bindra, D. (1974). A motivational view of learning, performance, and behaviour modification. *Psychological Review*, **8**, 199–213.

Burton, S. & Tiffany, S.T. (1994). Impact of alcohol intoxication on reactivity to smoking-related cues. Manuscript in preparation.

Burton, S.M., Drobes, D.J. & Tiffany, S.T. (1992). The manipulation of mood and smoking urges through imagery: evaluation of facial EMG activity. Paper presented at the annual meeting of the Midwestern Psychological Association, Chicago.

Cacioppo, J.T. & Tassinary, L.G. (Eds) (1990a). *Principles of Psychophysiology: Physical, Social and Inferential Elements*. New York: Cambridge University Press.

Cacioppo, J.T. & Tassinary, L.G. (1990b). Psychophysiology and psychophysiological inference. In J.T. Cacioppo & L.G. Tassinary (Eds), *Principles of Psychophysiology*, pp. 3–33. New York: Cambridge University Press.

Cepeda-Benito, A. & Tiffany, S.T. (1992). Effect of number of conditioning trials on the development of associative tolerance to morphine. *Psychopharmacology*, **109**, 172–176.

Cepeda-Benito, A. & Tiffany, S.T. (1994). The use of a dual-task procedure for the assessment of cognitive effort associated with smoking urges. Manuscript submitted for publication.

Childress, A.R., McLellan, A.T., Natale, M. & O'Brien, C.P. (1987). Mood states can illicit conditioned withdrawal and craving in opiate abuse patients. *NIDA Research Monographs*, **76**, 137–144.

Coles, M.G.H., Porges, S.W. & Donchin, E. (1986). *Psychophysiology: System, Process and Applications*. New York: Guilford.

Dafters, R. & Anderson, G. (1982). Conditioned tolerance to the tachycardia effect of ethanol in humans. *Psychopharmacology*, **78**, 365–367.

de Wit, H. & Chutaupe, M.A. (1993). Increased ethanol choice in social drinkers following ethanol preload. *Behavioural Pharmacology*, **4**, 29–36.

Diener, E. & Emmons, R.A. (1984). The independence of positive and negative affect. *Journal of Personality and Social Psychology*, **47**, 1105–1117.

Drobes, D.J. & Tiffany, S.T. (1994). Comparisons of smoking urges elicited through imagery and in vivo cue exposure. Manuscript submitted for publication.

Drummond, D.C. & Glautier, S. (1994). A controlled trial of cue exposure treatment in alcohol dependence. *Journal of Consulting and Clinical Psychology*, **62**, 809–817.

Ehrman, R., Ternes, J., O'Brien, C.P. & McLellan, A.T. (1992). Conditioned tolerance in human opiate addicts. *Psychopharmacology*, **108**, 218–224.

Elash, C.A., Tiffany, S.T. & Vrana, S.R. (1995). The manipulation of smoking urges through a brief imagery procedure: self-report, psychophysiological, and startle-probe responses. *Experimental and Clinical Psychopharmacology*, in press.

Everitt, B.S. & Dunn, G. (1991). *Applied Multivariate data Analysis*. London: Edward Arnold.

Glautier, S. & Drummond, D.C. (1994). Alcohol dependence and cue reactivity. *Journal of Studies on Alcohol*, **55**, 224–229.

Glautier, S., Drummond, C. & Remington, R. (1994). Alcohol as an unconditioned stimulus in human classical conditioning. *Psychopharmacology*, **116**, 360–368.

Goldberg, S.R. & Stolerman, I.P. (1986). *Behavioural Analysis of Drug Dependence*. London: Academic Press.

Goudie, A.J. & Demellweek, C. (1986). Conditioning factors in drug tolerance. In S.R. Goldberg & I.P. Stolerman (Eds), *Behavioral Analysis of Drug Dependence*, pp. 225–285. New York: Academic Press.

Hall, G. (1991). *Perceptual and Associative Learning*. Oxford: Clarendon Press.

Harris, J.D. (1943). Studies of non-associative factors inehrent in conditioning. *Comparative Psychological Monographs*, **18**, serial no. 1.

Hodgson, R., Rankin, H. & Stockwell, T. (1979). Alcohol dependence and the priming effect. *Behaviour Research and Therapy*, **17**, 379–387.

Holman, E.W. (1975). Some conditions for the dissociation of consummatory and instrumental behaviour in rats. *Learning and Motivation*, **6**, 358–366.

Jellinek, E.M. (1952). Current notes—phases of alcohol addiction. *Quarterly Journal of Studies on Alcohol*, **13**, 673–684.

Kaplan, R.F., Meyer, R.E. & Stroebel, C.F. (1983). Alcohol dependence and responsivity to an ethanol stimulus as predictors of alcohol consumption. *British Journal of Addictions*, **78**, 259–267.

Laberg, J.C. (1990). What is presented and what is prevented in cue exposure and response prevention with alcohol dependent subjects? *Addictive Behaviours*, **15**, 367–386.

Lacey, J.I. (1967). Somatic response patterning and stress: some revisions of activation theory. In M.H. Appley & R. Trumbull (Eds), *Psychological Stress: Issues in Research*. New York: Appleton Century Crofts.

Litman, G.K., Stapleton, J., Oppenheim, A.N., Peleg, M. & Jackson, P. (1983). Situations related to alcoholism relapse. *British Journal of Addiction*, **78**, 381–389.

Litt, M.D., Cooney, N.L., Kadden, R.M. & Gaupp, L. (1990). Reactivity to alcohol cues and induced moods in alcoholics. *Addictive Behaviours*, **15**, 137–146.

Ludwig, A.M., Wikler, A. & Stark, L.H. (1974). The first drink: psychobiological aspects of craving. *Archives of General Psychiatry*, **30**, 539–547.

Marlatt, G.A. & Gordon, J.R. (1980). Determinants of relapse: implications for the maintenance of behaviour change. In P.O. Davidson & S.M. Davison (Eds), *Behavioural Medicine: Changing Health Lifestyles*. New York: Bruner/Mazel.

Marlatt, G.A. & Rohsenow, D.J. (1980). Cognitive processes in alcohol use: expectancy and the balanced placebo design. In N.K. Mello (Ed.), *Advances in Substances Abuse*, Vol. 1. Greenwich, JAI Press.

Maude-Griffin, P.M. & Tiffany, S.T. (1994). Verbal and physiological manifestations of smoking urges produced through imagery: role of affect and smoking abstinence. Manuscript submitted for publication.
McCaul, M.E., Turkkan, J.S. & Stitzer, M.L. (1989a). Conditioned opponent responses: placebo challenge in alcoholic subjects. *Alcoholism: Clinical and Experimental Research*, **13**, 631–635.
McCaul, M.E., Turkkan, J.S. & Stitzer, M.L. (1989b). Psychophysiological effects of alcohol related stimuli: i. The role of stimulus intensity. *Alcoholism: Clinical and Experimental Research*, **13**, 386–391.
Meehl, P.E. (1971). High school yearbooks: a reply to Schwartz. *Journal of Abnormal Psychology*, **77**, 143–148.
Mintz, J., Boyd, G., Rose, J.E., Charuvastra, V.C. & Jarvik, M.E. (1985). Alcohol increases cigarette smoking: a laboratory demonstration. *Addictive Behaviours*, **10**, 203–207.
Naitoh, P. (1972). The effect of alcohol on the autonomic nervous system of humans: a psychophysiological approach. In B. Kissin and H. Begleiter (Eds), *The Biology of Alcoholism: Volume 2 Physiology and Behaviour*. New York: Plenum Press.
Nesselroade, J.R. & R.B. Cattell (Eds) (1988). *Handbook of Multivariate Experimental Psychology*, 2nd edn. New York: Plenum Press.
Newlin, D.B. (1985). The antagonistic placebo response to alcohol cues. *Alcoholism: Clinical and Experimental Research*, **9**, 411–416.
Newlin, D.B., Hotchkiss, B., Cox, W.M., Rauscher, F. & Li, T.K. (1989). Autonomic and subjective responses to alcohol stimuli with appropriate control stimuli. *Addictive Behaviours*, **14**, 625–630.
Nil, R., Buzzi, R. & Battig, K. (1984). Effects of single doses of alcohol and caffeine on cigarette smoke puffing behaviour. *Pharmacology, Biochemistry and Behaviour*, **20**, 583–590.
Pavlov, I.P. (1927). *Conditioned Reflexes*. New York: Dover Publications Inc. reprinted 1960.
Payne, T.J., Schare, M.L., Levis, D.J. & Colleti, G. (1991). Exposure to smoking-relevant cues: Effects on desire to smoke and topographical components of smoking behaviour. *Addictive Behaviours*, **16**, 467–479.
Pomerleau, O.F., Fertig, J., Baker, L. & Cooney, N. (1983). Reactivity to alcohol cues in alcoholics and non-alcoholics: implications for a stimulus control analysis of drinking. *Addictive Behaviours*, **8**, 1–10.
Powell, J., Bradley, B. & Gray, J. (1992). Classical conditioning and cognitive determinants of subjective craving for opiates: an investigation of their relative contributions. *British Journal of Addiction*, **87**, 1133–1144.
Powell, J., Gray, J.A., Bradley, B.P., Kasvikis, Y., Strang, J., Barrat, L. & Marks, I. (1990). The effects of exposure to drug-related cues in detoxified opiate addicts: a theoretical review and some new data. *Addictive Behaviours*, **15**, 339–345.
Rankin, H.J., Hodgson, R. & Stockwell, T. (1979). The concept of craving and its measurement. *Behaviour Research and Therapy*, **17**, 389–396.
Rescorla, R.A. (1966). Predictability and number of pairings in Pavlovian fear conditioning. *Psychonomic Science*, **4**, 383–384.
Rescorla, R.A. (1967). Pavlovian conditioning and its proper control procedures. *Psychological Review*, **74**, 71–80.
Rescorla, R.A. (1968). Probability of shock in the presence and absence of CS in fear conditioning. *Journal of Comparative and Physiological Psychology*, **66**, 1–5.
Rickard-Figueroa, K. & Zeichner, A. (1985). Assessment of smoking urge and its

concomitants under an environmental smoking cue manipulations. *Addictive Behaviours*, **10**, 249–256.

Robbins, S.J. & Ehrman, R.N. (1992). Designing studies of drug conditioning in humans. *Psychopharmacology*, **106**, 143–153.

Sherman, J.E., Zinser, M.C., Sideroff, S.I. & Baker, T.B. (1989). Subjective dimensions of heroin urges: influence of heroin-related and affectively negative stimuli. *Addictive Behaviours*, **14**, 611–623.

Siegel, S. (1983). Classical conditioning, drug tolerance and drug dependence. In Y. Israel, F.B. Glaser, H. Kalant, R.E. Popham, W. Schmidt & R.G. Smart (Eds), *Research Advances in Alcohol and Drug Problems*, Vol. 7, pp. 207–246. New York: Plenum Press.

Siegel, S. (1984). Pavlovian conditioning and heroin overdose: reports by overdose victims. *Bulletin of the Psychonomic Society*, **22**, 428–430.

Siegel, S. (1989). Pharmacological conditioning and drug effects. In A.J. Goudie & M.W. Emmett-Oglesby (Eds), *Psychoactive Drugs: Tolerance and Sensitization*. Clifton, NJ: Humana Press.

Singleton, E., Tiffany, S.T. & Henningfield, J.E. (1994). A questionnaire for the assessment of alcohol craving. Unpublished manuscript.

Stockwell, T.R., Hodgson, R.J., Rankin, H.J. & Taylor, C. (1982). Alcohol dependence, beliefs and the priming effect. *Behaviour Research and Therapy*, **20**, 513–522.

Tiffany, S.T. (1990). A cognitive model of drug urges and drug-use behaviour: role of automatic and non-automatic processes. *Psychological Review*, **97**, 147–168.

Tiffany, S.T. (1992). A critique of contemporary urge and craving research: Methodological, psychometric and theoretical issues. *Advances in Behaviour Research and Therapy*, **14**, 123–139.

Tiffany, S.T. & Drobes, D.J. (1990). Imagery and smoking urges: the manipulation of affective content. *Addictive Behaviours*, **15**, 531–539.

Tiffany, S.T. & Drobes, D.J. (1991). The development and initial validation of a questionnaire of smoking urges. *British Journal of Addiction*, **86**, 1467–1476.

Tiffany, S.T., Drobes, D.J. & Cepeda-Benito, A. (1992). Contribution of associative and non-associative processes to the development of morphine tolerance. *Psychopharmacology*, **109**, 185–190.

Tiffany, S.T., Maude-Griffin, P.M. & Drobes, D.J. (1991). The effect of inter-dose interval on the development of associative and non-associative tolerance. *Behavioral Neuroscience*, **105**, 49–61.

Tiffany, S.T., Singleton, E., Haertzen, C.A. & Henningfield, J.E. (1993). The development and initial validation of a cocaine craving questionnaire. *Drug and Alcohol Dependence*, **34**, 19–28.

Tiffany, S.T., Field, L., Singleton, E., Haertzen, C. & Henningfield, J.E. (1994). The development of a heroin craving questionnaire. Manuscript in preparation.

Toates, F.M. (1986). *Motivational Systems*. New York: Cambridge University Press.

Turkkan, J.S. (1989). Classical conditioning: the new hegemony. *Behavioural and Brain Sciences*, **12**, 121–179.

Wagner, A.R. & Brandon, S.E. (1989). Evolution of a structured connectionist model of Pavlovian conditioning (AESOP). In S.B. Klein & R.R. Mowrer (Eds), *Contemporary Learning Theories: Pavlovian Conditioning and the Status of Traditional Learning Theory*. Hillsdale, NJ: Lawrence Erlbaum.

Watson, D., Clark, L.A. & Tellegen, A. (1988). Development and validation of brief measures of positive and negative affect: the PANAS scales. *Journal of Personality and Social Psychology*, **54**, 1063–1070.

Wetter, D.W., Brandon, T.H. & Baker, T.B. (1992). The relation of affective processing measures and smoking motivation indices among college-age smokers. *Advanced Behaviour Research and Therapy*, **14**, 169–193.

Wickens, D.D. & Wickens, C.D. (1942). Some factors related to pseudoconditioning. *Journal of Experimental Psychology*, **31**, 518–526.

Woodward, J.W. & Goldstein, M.S. (1977). Communication deviance in the families of schizophrenics: a comment on the misuses of analysis of covariance. *Science*, **197**, 1097.

Young, A.M. & Goudie, A.J. (in press). Adaptive processes regulating tolerance to behavioral effects of drugs. In F.E. Bloom & D.J. Kupfer (Eds), *Psychopharmacology: The Fourth Generation of Progress*. New York: Raven Press.

Zappulla, R.A., LeFever, F.F., Jaeger, J. & Bilder, R. (Eds) (1991). *Windows on the Brain: Neuropsychology's Technological Frontiers*, Vol. 620. New York: The New York Academy of Sciences.

CHAPTER 5

Individual differences and cue reactivity

Vaughan W. Rees and
Nick Heather[†]

The identification of factors which result in individual variation, and how those factors influence psychological performance, now occupies an important place in modern psychology. Personality, psychological traits, genetic or familial variables, sex and age, among others, have received attention as candidates which contribute to psychological heterogeneity. The study of drug cue reactivity is an area where identification and explanation of factors that contribute to individual variability can be of great potential benefit, by explaining discrepancies in previous research and assisting in the development of a more complete account of the phenomenon.

The emphasis in cue reactivity research has focused on understanding the way in which group factors come to produce changes in responsivity to drug stimuli. The factors that have been most thoroughly investigated are derived largely from the dominant conditioning models of drug cue reactivity (Wikler, 1965; Siegel, 1983; Stewart, de Wit & Eikelboom, 1984). Predictions of these models are, by their nature, oriented toward the examination of group differences. It might be argued that the investigation of a new and challenging phenomenon should logically commence in such a fashion, in order to establish critical experimental parameters. Attainment of further knowledge will be accelerated with the findings gained from tests of the major theoretically derived hypotheses. Therefore it is likely that a group, or nomothetic, approach is an appropriate one for testing the key conditioning-based hypotheses of cue reactivity. Certainly, this approach has yielded much data which have been moderately successful in explaining basic reactivity phenomena (see Drummond, Cooper & Glautier, 1990), and addressing the clinical useful-

*University of New South Wales, Sydney, Australia, and [†]Northern Regional Alcohol and Drug Service, Newcastle-upon-Tyne, UK.

Addictive Behaviour: Cue Exposure Theory and Practice.
Edited by D.C. Drummond, S.T. Tiffany, S. Glautier and B. Remington.
© 1995 John Wiley & Sons Ltd.

ness of cue exposure (Monti et al., 1993b). But it appears that the picture is far from complete. We seem to be some way yet from identifying specifically how, for example, cue reactivity is developed, what determines level and type of responsivity and how individual characteristics influence responsivity to drug cues.

As in other areas of psychological research, the question arises as to why some individuals are responsive to certain manipulations while others are not. For example, in several cue reactivity studies it has been reported that a large proportion of subjects showed little or no response to a cue exposure manipulation. Childress, McLellan & O'Brien (1986) reported that half of their sample of methadone-maintained subjects did not experience craving in response to heroin-related cues. One-third of subjects did not show changes on physiological measures. Potentially, methadone maintenance might diminish cue reactivity. However, Powell, Bradley & Gray (1992) reported that over one-third of their sample of detoxified opiate users did not experience increases in cue-elicited craving. On other measures of subjective reactivity, up to two-thirds of subjects failed to show responses to drug cues. Reactivity to alcohol-related cues appears to show similar response patterns. Almost one-third of alcohol-dependent subjects have failed to show cue-specific increases in desire, and a similar proportion did not experience increases in salivation when presented with alcohol-related cues (Monti et al., 1993a).

Furthermore, it is not unreasonable to assume that, within the subjects who do show reactivity to drug cues, there is considerable variability in the magnitude of reactivity. One important contribution that individual differences can provide to the field of cue reactivity is recognition that cue reactivity might not be an all-or-none phenomenon, but rather one of varying levels of responsivity between individuals. Moreover, the direction of the cue-elicited response might differ between individuals. Recent reports have shown both increased and decreased reactivity on the same measure, within the same paradigm (Greeley, Swift & Heather, 1993). Thus, the degree as well as the direction of reactivity might differ between individuals. The nature of reactivity should be predictable by theoretically determined factors, which must include individual difference variables. Identifying those variables will surely enhance explanatory models of cue reactivity.

The application of individual difference research techniques in other areas of addiction research is relatively well established. In particular, exploration of genetic and familial factors that potentially predispose an individual to drug abuse has received considerable attention (e.g. Cloninger, 1987). Although individual differences have seldom been considered specifically in studies of cue reactivity, there is limited evidence that certain factors might predict *a priori* the nature of cue-elicited responses to drug stimuli. These factors include measures of dependence, social learning constructs, affective states, personality characteristics and familial history of drug and alcohol abuse. The present chapter will consider the influence of these factors on individual variability in cue reactivity.

CUE REACTIVITY AND LEVEL OF DEPENDENCE

Conditioning models of cue reactivity hypothesize that response magnitude will be greatest in those whose drug-use histories involve greater quantity and frequency of consumption. It would be predicted on this basis that drug-dependent individuals will show greater reactivity than non-dependent individuals, and that severity of dependence will be positively related to magnitude of reactivity (e.g. Heather & Greeley, 1990). Using level of dependence as an individual difference measure, the magnitude of subjective and physiological cue reactivity should be predictable.

Because reactivity to drug cues is closely associated with drug dependence, the phenomenon has been more thoroughly investigated in subjects with higher dependence. However, assessment of cue reactivity in non-dependent drug users might not only help to identify fundamental differences between dependent and non-dependent users, but could potentially provide other information such as the relationship between cue reactivity and level of prior drug consumption. Reactivity in non-dependent individuals is of little clinical significance and therefore such individuals are usually only included as controls. In studies of opiate- and cocaine-related cue reactivity, control subjects are drug naive (e.g. Ehrman et al., 1992). However, with studies of alcohol-related cue reactivity, it is possible to recruit control subjects who have drinking experience but are without a history of prolonged heavy or problem drinking. Therefore, most of the relevant evidence in this area comes from studies of alcohol-related cue reactivity.

Physiological reactivity and self-reports of cue-elicited urges/desires will be considered separately to highlight differences in findings from these general response domains.

Level of Dependence and Physiological Reactivity

Although alcohol cue-specific responses typically are not observed on all physiological measures, there is a clear trend for greater physiological reactivity in subjects with higher levels of dependence. Compared with non-dependent drinkers, alcohol-dependent individuals have been found to show greater responsivity to alcohol cues on measures of skin conductance (Kaplan, Meyer & Stroebel, 1983; Kaplan et al., 1985), heart rate (Kaplan et al., 1985; McCusker & Brown, 1991), salivation (McCusker & Brown, 1991; Monti et al., 1987), and swallowing (Pomerleau et al., 1983). Subjective measures of arousal (McCusker & Brown, 1991) and anxiety (Abrams et al., 1991; McCusker & Brown, 1991) have been found to be greater in dependent drinkers, suggesting possible cue-elicited increases in autonomic reactivity in those subjects. In a study of drinkers not in treatment, Greeley et al. (1993) reported that heavy drinkers showed a differing pattern of heart rate response to successive alcohol cue exposures compared to light drinkers. One novel study found that dependent drinkers showed greater and more rapid glucose and insulin responses after exposure to placebo beverage cues, compared with non-dependent controls (Dolinsky et al., 1987). However, some failures to observe greater physiological reactivity in dependent drinkers have been reported. Although dependent and non-dependent drinkers experienced significant cue-elicited increases in heart rate and skin conductance, these measures did not differ between groups (Abrams et al., 1991; Dolinsky et al., 1987).

These results suggest that physiological reactivity is heavily influenced by level of dependence. Although there were various physiological measures that failed to distinguish dependent and non-dependent subjects in the studies cited above, in no case did non-dependent subjects show greater physiological reactivity to alcohol cues. In general, dependent subjects showed a pattern of greater reactivity to alcohol cues, supporting predictions of conditioning models on the influence of dependence on cue reactivity.

Level of Dependence and Self-Reported Urge Reactivity

Research on urge reactivity with light and social drinkers suggests that self-reported urges are readily elicited in this group by exposure to alcohol-related cues. However, there is no clear consensus among studies as to the role of level of dependence on the cue-elicited urge response. Contrary to predictions derived from conditioning theory and despite the positive findings regarding level of dependence and physiological reactivity, few studies have shown that cue-elicited urge to drink is greater in heavy drinkers than light drinkers. Kaplan, Meyer & Stroebel (1983) observed differing levels of cue-elicited urge between dependent drinkers and normal drinking controls. As predicted, the strongest desire was observed in dependent drinkers compared with social drinkers. However, desire to drink in the dependent drinkers was strongly related to the expectation of receiving alcohol. Although suggestive, evidence of differential urge responding between dependent and non-dependent drinkers in this study could have been confounded by elements of an interoceptive alcohol cue which only half of the subjects received. Those subjects who received alcohol prior to cue exposure had greater self-reported urges overall. Pomerleau et al. (1983) reported higher craving in dependent drinkers compared with non-dependent controls after exposure to alcohol beverage sight and smell cues. Greater desire in alcohol abusers was also observed by Abrams et al. (1991) who exposed alcohol abusers and social drinkers to simulated high-risk relapse situations. Urge to drink was higher in the alcohol abuser group in both alcohol-specific and general social role play situations. In a study of heavy and light drinkers, Greeley et al. (1993) found that self-reported desire ratings clearly differed according to level of dependence. Of interest is the pattern of response over time. The response of heavy drinkers to successive exposures to alcohol sight, smell and taste cues was characterized by a steady increase. In comparison, light drinkers reported an initial increase in desire which diminished over the course of exposures.

Other studies have failed to demonstrate a clear influence of alcohol dependence on cue-elicited desire. Although both dependent and non-dependent drinkers have reported significant increases in cue-elicited desire, several studies have found no difference in urge reactivity between groups (Corty, O'Brien & Mann, 1988; Dolinsky et al., 1987; Kaplan et al., 1985; Monti et al., 1987). Cooney et al. (1987) found that desire to drink was rated as *greater* by non-dependent subjects compared with dependent drinkers, although both groups showed increased self-reported urge to drink in response to alcohol cues.

Unlike physiological reactivity, there is only limited evidence to confirm that self-reported urge responding is greater in alcohol-dependent subjects. There might be several reasons for this. Firstly, cue-elicited desire might indeed be relatively strong even in social drinkers. If this desire is the result of conditioning, it might be concluded that drug urges quickly reach an asymptotic level, since social drinkers have numerous opportunities to experience alcohol and cue pairings. This could result in similar urge reports from both severely dependent subjects and social drinkers. What these urge responses represent in terms of motivational significance for drinking behaviour for heavy and light users, respectively, would require clarification. Secondly, it has been suggested that alcohol-dependent subjects operate on a different "metric" to non-dependent subjects when rating their urges to drink (e.g. Cooney et al., 1987). It is not unreasonable to expect that individuals who have experienced severe manifestations of alcohol dependence will interpret urges, especially in a laboratory situation, differently to those who have never been dependent. In response to experimental cue exposure, individuals who are dependent on alcohol might rate desire more conservatively, reflecting perhaps a comparison between the present state and more extreme desires experienced in real life. Thirdly, according to Wise (1988), drug urges may arise from separate neural centres for positive and negative reinforcement. While positive incentive urges would be observed in both dependent and non-dependent drinkers, urges arising from the negative reinforcement system would be expected to be more frequently observed in dependent drinkers, whose drinking would often be prompted by symptoms of withdrawal. If stimuli that represent positive reinforcement are presented, both dependent and non-dependent subjects might experience similar levels of urge activation.

Finally, differential histories of drug cue pairings between individuals might result in conditioned drug stimulus complexes that are highly idiosyncratic. Presentation of a powerful drug cue might result in reactivity for some individuals only if a relevant occasion-setting stimulus is also present. Occasion setters signal that other cues will be reinforced, although they are not associated with direct elicitation of conditioned drug responses (Holland, 1983). Occasion setters possibly differ widely between individuals, and depending on the presence or absence of such a stimulus in the cue exposure paradigm, some individuals may fail to experience reactivity to an otherwise potent cue. Potentially, certain emotional and motivational states could act as occasion-setting stimuli for drug cues, such that the additional presence of depression, anxiety, or a state of withdrawal might be necessary for some individuals to react to drug cues (see Greeley & Ryan, Chapter 6). Corty, O'Brien & Mann (1988) have argued that both expectancy of receiving alcohol and the physical setting are important in the elicitation of alcohol-related cue reactivity. In situations where alcohol is obviously unavailable, or where the physical surroundings do not reflect a real drinking or drug-use environment, cue reactivity in heavier users might be diminished.

Relationship between Measures of Dependence and Cue Reactivity

Attempts to relate severity of dependence directly to magnitude of reactivity have produced inconsistent findings in different response domains.

Although methods of measuring dependence differ, this variable provides a useful index of "conditioning experience".

Direct measures of dependence

By direct measures of dependence we mean instruments that have been developed specifically to measure drug dependence (e.g. Severity of Alcohol Dependence Questionnaire (SADQ), Stockwell et al., 1979; Alcohol Dependence Scale (ADS), Skinner & Allen, 1982). As predicted by a conditioning model of cue reactivity, correlations between level of alcohol dependence and urge and salivatory cue reactivity have been observed (Rohsenow et al., 1992). However, other studies have obtained correlations between dependence and only urge reactivity (Monti et al., 1987), or only salivatory reactivity (McCusker & Brown, 1991), while another found no correlation between either measure (Monti et al., 1993a). However, Monti et al. (1993a) found that urge "reactors" (subjects who showed greater responses to alcohol cues than neutral cues) were more dependent than urge "non-reactors". Salivatory reactors were also more dependent, and consumed more drinks per day and had less days of abstinence than salivatory non-reactors. In a study of smoking cue reactivity, Payne et al. (1991) found correlations between nicotine dependence and topographical measures of smoking behaviour. Direct correlation between dependence and desire was, however, not significant.

Indirect measures of dependence

Other studies have used measures such as quantity of consumption and duration of use as indices of dependence. Number of heavy drinking days has been found to correlate with cue-elicited change in skin conductance, but not desire to drink (Kaplan et al., 1985). In a study of non-dependent drinkers, number of drinks consumed per week correlated with both cue-elicited desire to drink and heart rate (White & Staiger, 1991). Measures based upon period of abuse have proved to be unsuccessful in relating dependence with reactivity. McCusker & Brown (1991) found that number of years of drinking was not associated with either desire or salivatory reactivity. In a study of reactivity to opiate cues, Powell et al. (1990) found that number of years of addiction and severity of use in the last month were not related to cue-elicited craving. However, severity of withdrawal symptoms and use of drugs to relieve withdrawal, arguably better indices of opiate dependence, were significantly correlated with cue-elicited craving. Level of cue-elicited craving was found to correlate with severity of prior alcohol withdrawal symptoms by Ludwig, Wikler & Stark (1974).

In a study of reactivity to an alcohol priming dose, Hodgson, Rankin & Stockwell (1979) found that ratings of moderate or severe alcohol dependence by a psychiatrist correlated with urge to drink after the consumption of a priming dose of alcohol. However, this might have been due to pharmacological effects rather than reactivity to the sensory cues provided by the alcoholic beverage (see Drummond, Cooper & Glautier, 1990).

These results are difficult to interpret. While direct and indirect measures of dependence have been associated with both urge and physiological reactivity, some studies have failed to observe such relationships. This could be due to differences in factors such as subject samples, experimental procedure, cue types and method of assessing dependence. Direct measures of dependence appear to be no more successful than indirect measures in relating dependence with magnitude of cue reactivity.

In many studies the subject sample has been restricted to subjects with relatively severe dependence. Correlational analysis would favour data drawn from samples with wide variability in dependence scores (e.g. White & Staiger, 1991). For this purpose, inclusion of light drinkers and non-drinkers might increase the range of dependence scores, and the likelihood of observing a significant relationship between dependence and cue reactivity. This might help to explain failures to show a positive relationship between level of dependence and reactivity. Overall, the available evidence suggests that level of dependence does influence individual patterns of cue reactivity, but further research is required to establish the precise function of this factor.

SOCIAL LEARNING CONSTRUCTS

Potentially important sources of individual variability in cue reactivity are those factors known to influence individual drug-taking behaviour, such as the social learning constructs of outcome and self-efficacy expectancies. Individuals who have low self-efficacy, and high positive expectancies for the effects of drug use, are predicted to show greater desire for drug use and be at greater risk for relapse (Marlatt & Gordon, 1985). Because exposure to drug cues represents a high-risk situation, cue reactivity would be expected to be greater in individuals who have more positive outcome expectancies and lower self-efficacy.

Positive outcome expectancies for alcohol consumption have been associated with increased physiological and subjective cue reactivity in several studies. Cooney et al. (1984) found that salivatory reactivity correlated with positive outcome expectancies for the taste of the beverage and the pleasurable and stimulating effects of alcohol. However, urge reactivity was not related to positive outcome expectancies. A further study (Cooney et al., 1987) found that urge to drink was correlated with positive expectancies for the taste and feeling of alcohol. Enjoyment of the sight and the smell of an alcohol cue has been observed to correlate highly with salivatory and urge reactivity (see Rohsenow et al., 1992). Positive expectancies of sexual enhancement, power/aggression, social expressiveness and tension reduction correlated significantly with salivatory reactivity, but only expectancy of increased power/aggression correlated with urge reactivity in studies reported by Rohsenow et al. (1992).

Considering the importance of the self-efficacy construct in addictive behaviour, this variable has received surprisingly little attention as a predictor for cue reactivity. Consistent with Marlatt & Gordon's (1985) social learning model of relapse, Greeley, Swift & Heather (1992) reported strong negative correlations between subjects' cue-elicited desire for alcohol and self-reported efficacy expectancies of being able to resist drinking in "positive social situations" and while experiencing "urges and temptations" to drink. Questions on these subscales of the Situational Confidence Questionnaire (SCQ-39) (Annis & Graham, 1988) make reference to actual drinking situations, where alcohol cues are present. Hence, it is understandable that those subjects who experienced strongest urge reactivity would score lower on these scales. In a study of cue-elicited positive and "negative" urges (desire *not* to drink), Greeley, Swift & Heather (1993) found that, of eight demographic and alcohol-use measures, only self-efficacy differentiated subjects reporting positive desire from those reporting negative desire. Subjects who reported positive desires were found to have lower self-efficacy than those who reported negative desires.

These findings suggest that self-efficacy and positive outcome expectancies are important predictors of reactivity, particularly cue-elicited urges. Evidence for their influence on physiological reactivity is less clear. Further use of these constructs in studies of cue reactivity may help not only to explain individual variability in urge reactivity, but to further explain the way in which social learning constructs mediate drug urges.

AFFECTIVE STATES AND CUE REACTIVITY

Pre-existing affective states might also influence individual differences in responsivity. High levels of depression, anxiety and stress are thought to play an important role in initiating and maintaining drug use (Marlatt & Gordon, 1985). An appetitive motivational model of drug use predicts that negative mood states should increase the incentive value of some drugs, and make the expected effects of the drug more salient (Stewart, de Wit & Eikelboom, 1984). Baker, Morse & Sherman (1987) have proposed an affective-motivational model of drug use, in which urges are elicited by activation of either of two separate urge networks. Both positive and negative mood states can increase urges, and negative moods are thought to be particularly potent elicitors of urges during withdrawal because of the increased incentive value of the drug at this time. On the basis of the common predictions of these models, it would be expected that cue reactivity will be greatest in those individuals who have salient affective states at the time of exposure.

In two studies of alcohol-related cue reactivity which measured depression (see Rohsenow et al., 1992), significant correlations were observed between depression and urge reactivity, but not with salivatory reactivity. In support of this finding, Greeley, Swift & Heather (1992) found that cue-elicited desire for alcohol was predicted by subjects' level of depressed affect and mean daily alcohol consumption. These variables accounted for a significant 40% of the variance in self-reported desire for alcohol. Litt et al. (1990) also found that negative mood was related to enhanced desire to drink, but this was not specific to alcohol cue presentation. Level of anxiety prior to alcohol cue exposure was found to correlate with cue-elicited urge (Cooney et al., 1987), further supporting the influence of negative affective states as predictors of cue-elicited urges. Negative mood states have also been found to account for cue-elicited urges in opiate users (Sherman et al., 1989). Feelings of boredom, anxiety and anger were strongly related to desire when heroin-related cues were present.

These findings point to the importance of affective states, particularly negative ones, in influencing individual patterns of urge reactivity. This is consistent with theoretical models of drug urges (e.g. Marlatt & Gordon, 1985; Baker, Morse & Sherman, 1987). Although affective states are not generally associated with physiological reactivity, Rohsenow et al. (1992) have reported that salivatory reactors (subjects who reacted more strongly to alcohol cues than a control cue) were found to have higher depression scores than salivatory non-reactors. This would indicate that affective states influence not only urges, but possibly physiological reactivity as well.

DIFFERENTIAL CUE REACTIVITY IN RELAPSERS AND QUITTERS

Studies of smoking cue reactivity have found that reactivity in individuals who quit differs from those who relapse to smoking. Abrams et al. (1988) exposed groups of abstinent, relapsed and non-smokers to smoking cues in the form of a confederate smoker. Relapsed smokers were found to show increased heart rate and urge reactivity, and were significantly more anxious after cue exposure. Abstinent smokers did not differ from non-smokers. Because differences in reactivity might have been due to current smoking status, a further, prospective study by Abrams et al. (1988) was performed which measured cue reactivity prior to assignment to a smoking cessation programme. Those subjects who were successful in quitting were found to have significantly reduced heart rate and anxiety responses following exposure to cues compared with relapsers before treatment. A further analysis of these data by Niaura et al. (1989) examined the cardiac response to nicotine cues over the first nine heart beats after stimulus onset, thus providing a more sensitive index of cue-elicited responsivity. Relapsed smokers were differentiated from quitters on this measure, with a significant lengthening in inter-beat interval among the relapsers.

These preliminary findings point to a potentially important association between cue reactivity and individual susceptibility to relapse. It is not clear which factors underlie the greater responsivity in individuals who are more likely to relapse. Measures of dependence, years of smoking and number of cigarettes smoked daily before treatment were similar between groups. Furthermore, observer-rated behavioural skill in the presence of cues was similar for each group. Nevertheless, these studies suggest that ability to abstain from smoking, and perhaps other drug use, is related in some way to individual variability in cue reactivity.

FAMILIAL AND PERSONALITY FACTORS IN CUE REACTIVITY

A substantial literature supports the involvement of genetic (see Cotton, 1979) and personality (e.g. Cloninger, 1987; see also Tarter, Alterman & Edwards, 1985) factors in vulnerability to alcohol abuse. Although the way in which genetic and personality factors influence drug abuse behaviour is far from clear, there is limited evidence that these "high-risk" factors are associated with enhanced drug cue associative learning and responding. This section will consider how such factors influence individual differences in cue reactivity, and how drug cue associative learning might relate to vulnerability to drug and alcohol abuse.

Personality and Cue Reactivity

Personality has been considered as a mediating variable between inherited factors and actual drug-use behaviour. How this mediation occurs is obviously complex, but conditioning and social learning factors are likely to play an important role. For example, Cloninger's (1987) proposed "high-risk" personality types have their physiological bases in three distinct neural systems which differ in their responses to novel, appetitive and aversive stimuli. These genetically determined neural structures are thought to allow for enhanced associative learning of drug effects. If this is so, it would be expected that individuals with high-risk personality types show signs of enhanced drug-related conditioning. This might be evident in studies of drug cue reactivity both before and after the onset of alcohol abuse. Unfortunately, no cue reactivity studies have investigated whether individuals with "high-risk" personality or temperaments, using, for example, Cloninger's classification system, are more susceptible to drug-related conditioning.

However, individuals who are more susceptible to general conditioning processes may also develop more powerful drug cue associations, resulting in potentially greater drug cue reactivity. Eysenck's (1967) theory of personality makes specific predictions regarding individual conditioning potential among certain personality types. Introverts are presumed to easily acquire conditioned responses due to a higher level of cortical excitation, thus enhancing formation of excitatory associative links. In contrast, the cortical inhibition of extroverts results in reduced potential to develop excitatory conditioned responses. Neuroticism, attributable to elevated and labile limbic and autonomic activity, is thought to enhance conditioning potential in both introverts and extroverts (Eysenck, 1967).

Evidence from studies of cue reactivity

Evidence from recent studies of alcohol- and opiate-related cue reactivity lends preliminary support for the involvement of Eysenck's personality dimensions in determining individual patterns of cue responsivity. McCusker & Brown (1991) observed significant negative correlations between extroversion and cue-elicited salivation, arousal and anxiety in a sample of dependent drinkers. That is, subjects who were more introverted experienced greater cue-elicited reactivity. Furthermore neuroticism correlated significantly with salivatory reactivity. The extroversion and neuroticism dimensions accounted for larger proportions of the variance observed on measures of salivation and arousal than measures of physical dependence or drinking history, measures which traditional conditioning models predict to be highly correlated with cue reactivity. Assuming that reactivity to alcohol cues is the result of Pavlovian processes, McCusker & Brown's (1991) results are consistent with Eysenck's conditionability hypothesis. Individuals high on neuroticism and low on extroversion (introverts) were found to be more reactive to alcohol-related cues, suggesting that conditioning to such cues is more complete in that group.

Further hypotheses regarding individual variability in cue reactivity can be derived from Gray's (1970) modification of Eysenck's model, again based on principles of conditioning. Gray has proposed that introverts are more susceptible to punishment because of their reduced ability to dampen the effects of stimulation, owing to higher arousal. Conditioning will be enhanced in introverts when aversive reinforcement (i.e. punishment) is used, whereas extroverts are more sensitive to appetitive reinforcement (i.e. reward). Therefore, according to Gray, introverts are not necessarily more conditionable (cf. Eysenck, 1967), but are more sensitive to punishment.

Powell et al. (1990) reported findings from detoxified opiate users, using extroversion and neuroticism as predictors of cue-elicited craving. It was predicted that, if cue-elicited craving resulted from conditioning to both appetitive and aversive drug cues, reactivity would be associated equally with extroversion and introversion, producing no net effect. Because neuroticism is considered to enhance conditioning in both extroverts and introverts, reactivity should be greater in individuals who have high neuroticism. Consistent with these predictions, no correlation was observed between extroversion and cue-elicited craving, and neuroticism correlated moderately with craving. A further study (Powell, Bradley & Gray, 1992) also observed a significant positive correlation between neuroticism and cue-elicited craving.

Gray (1975) has argued that impulsive[1] individuals have increased sensitivity to conditioned reward signals, and will be more likely to show appetitive behavioural responses to cues associated with rewarding outcomes. In relation to drug cues, Powell, Bradley and Gray (1992) predicted that impulsive individuals would react with greater craving to drug cues. Impulsivity was found to correlate significantly with cue-elicited craving. Further analysis revealed that this relationship was mediated by positive outcome expectancies, possibly because highly impulsive individuals have increased sensitivity to conditioned signals for reward and thereby possess greater positive expectancies of drug effects. Powell, Bradley & Gray (1992) suggest that the relationship between neuroticism and craving is due to greater sensitivity to withdrawal and aversive physical symptoms in those subjects, and the negative reinforcement (and hence positive outcome expectancies) that opiate cues represent.

As the work of Powell and colleagues suggests, personality, as well as other measures of individual differences, has the potential to assist in the elucidation of general mechanisms of reactivity, such as the aversive/appetitive basis of conditioned craving responses. Further research using personality constructs as predictors of cue reactivity appears to be very much warranted. These studies provide preliminary support for a model of enhanced conditioning to drug cues in neurotic, introverted and impulsive individuals. It is interesting that these same personality constructs have been associated with alcohol and drug abuse. Neuroticism and introversion are high in opiate and polydrug abusers (Gossop & Eysenck, 1980) and have also been linked with severity of alcohol dependence (Rankin, Stockwell & Hodgson, 1982). Indeed, Tarter et al.'s (1985) high-risk temperament trait "emotionality" and Cloninger's (1987) dimension of "harm avoidance" have a close resemblance with the introverted–neurotic type hypothesized by Gray (1970, 1975) to be susceptible to conditioning.

Familial Factors and Cue Reactivity

Conditioned or learned responses that contribute to drug-use problems might be enhanced when an individual has a family history of substance abuse problems. The evidence for enhanced learning of responses to drug cues is limited, but studies by Newlin (1985) and Walitzer & Sher (1990) suggest that individuals who, by virtue of family history are at higher risk for drug abuse problems, might react differently to individuals without such a history. Administration of placebo has been shown to evoke antagonistic autonomic responses in subjects who had previously received alcohol in the presence of distinctive environmental cues (Newlin, 1986). Newlin (1986) observed a decrease in pulse transit time and skin temperature, which usually are increased markedly by alcohol consumption, after consumption of the placebo. The antagonistic placebo response is probably a compensatory conditioned response to drug cues (e.g. Siegel, 1983). Newlin (1985) found that offspring of alcoholic fathers experienced greater antagonistic heart rate responses compared to normal controls. Offspring of alcoholics also reported slightly greater subjective intoxication than controls. However, other autonomic measures, such as pulse transit time, finger pulse amplitude and general motor activity, failed to distinguish the two groups.

The results provide tentative evidence for a role for familial factors in cue reactivity. Precisely how this apparent predisposition for drug cue responding is derived is not known. It is tempting to conclude that off-spring of problem drinkers possess innate mechanisms that enhance conditioning to drug cues, which in turn, contribute to problem drinking itself. Newlin (1985) provides one proposed mechanism for this rapid progression, using conditioned drug tolerance as a contributing mechanism. The phenomenon of drug tolerance has been shown to be mediated, at least in part, by Pavlovian processes (Siegel, 1983). Drug antagonistic responses that are elicited by conditioned cues enable individuals to tolerate the effects of alcohol better, compared to situations where drug cues are not available. While the relationship between tolerance and alcohol dependence is not a simple one, the two phenomena are often observed together and correlate strongly (see Cappell & Le Blanc, 1982). One simple proposed relationship between tolerance and dependence suggests that tolerant individuals have the capacity to consume a greater quantity of drug, thus accelerating dependence problems (Siegel, 1983). This might apply to those whose tolerance is acquired through accelerated conditioning processes.

Furthermore, the greater subjective intoxication after placebo observed by Newlin (1985) might be related to the finding that problem drinkers are less able to discriminate blood alcohol level compared with controls (Lipscomb & Nathan, 1980). Offspring of problem drinkers are less able to determine subjectively level of actual intoxication than controls (Schuckit, 1980, 1984). Reduced sensitivity to the effects of intoxication might constitute one way in which patterns of problem drinking are developed in persons with familial susceptibility.

Walitzer & Sher (1990) explored the role of familial history of drinking problems in cue reactivity. While measures of salivation and desire to drink were significantly greater in response to an alcohol cue compared to a control cue for the sample as a whole, no differences between high-risk and low-risk subjects were observed in response to the alcohol cue. However, some evidence for differential physiological responding between the two groups was obtained. High-risk subjects showed greater salivatory responses at baseline. It is possible that this was due to the effects of a small priming dose administered prior to the cue exposure procedure. Although not argued explicitly by the authors, it might be possible that the alcohol priming dose elicited differential responsivity between the two groups owing to its interoceptive cue properties (e.g. Ludwig, Wikler & Stark, 1974). High-risk subjects also showed greater electromyographic and skin temperature cue reactivity activity than control subjects, although this response was not specific to the alcoholic beverage cue. The results, while largely negative, suggest that high-risk individuals might exhibit a pattern of autonomic reactivity that differentiates them from normal controls. Although this reactivity was not alcohol specific, the pattern of responses was similar to that observed in problem drinkers (Kaplan et al., 1985), and might subserve processes which enable greater conditioning to alcohol cues in the future.

Although probably a minor source of individual variability in studies of cue reactivity, familial factors could potentially allow enhanced learning to drug cues. Despite the relatively small effects observed in these studies, further work in this area might be fruitful, particularly if familial factors are employed in conjunction with measures of high-risk personality.

CONCLUSION

There is little doubt that individual differences contribute greatly to the magnitude, and possibly even the type, of cue reactivity. The way in which the individual difference measures reviewed here contribute to variation in cue reactivity is mainly consistent with existing theoretical models of cue reactivity. Conditioning models of reactivity which predict greater responsivity in more heavily dependent individuals have good utility in explaining differences in magnitude of physiological reactivity between individuals, based upon level of dependence. However, cue-elicited drugs do not generally conform to this prediction, and the involvement of additional explanatory factors must be sought. The social learning constructs of self-efficacy and positive outcome expectancies might be more useful in predicting individual patterns of urge reactivity. The usefulness of these constructs in explaining subjective responses to drug use has been widely recognized, but perhaps poorly used as an explanation for varying patterns of cue reactivity. Affective states have also been linked in theoretical models with urge elicitation, but again, have been poorly utilized as predictors of reactivity. The available evidence suggests that pre-existing affective states have a strong bearing on the elicitation of urges. Further research should aim to develop existing models of mood-mediated urges. The role of affective states as occasion-setting stimuli probably also deserves further attention. Finally, "high-risk" familial and personality factors might also play a role in determining individual responsivity to drug cues. While these factors probably do not result in wide individual variation within cue reactivity studies, they are extremely important as variables that may enhance individual susceptibility to acquire conditioned responses to drug cues. This is an area that deserves greater attention, as methodology refined in studies of cue reactivity can be used to explore the possible learning-mediated relationship between inherited high-risk factors and drug abuse.

NOTE

1. Impulsiveness was initially conceived as one of several intercorrelated traits of which extroversion is comprised (Eysenck, 1967). Further work (Eysenck et al., 1985) has established that this trait is better regarded as aligned with psychoticism, and is often referred to as impulsivity.

REFERENCES

Abrams, D.B., Monti, P.M., Carey, K.B., Pinto, R.P. & Jacobus, S.I. (1988). Reactivity to smoking cues and relapse: two studies of discriminant validity. *Behaviour Research and Therapy*, **26**, 225–233.

Abrams, D.B., Binkoff, J.A., Zwick, W.R., Liepman, M.R., Nirenberg, T.D., Munroe, S.M. & Monti, P.M. (1991). Alcohol abusers' and social drinkers' responses to alcohol-relevant and general situations. *Journal of Studies on Alcohol*, **52**, 409–414.

Annis, H.M. & Graham, J.M. (1988). *Situational Confidence Questionnaire (SCQ) User's Guide*. Toronto: Addiction Research Foundation.

Baker, T.B., Morse, E. & Sherman, J.E. (1987). The motivation to use drugs: a psychobiological analysis of urges. In P.C. Rivers (Ed.), *Nebraska Symposium on Motivation: Alcohol Use and Abuse*, pp. 257–283. Lincoln, NB: University of Nebraska Press.

Cappell, H. & Le Blanc, A.E. (1982). Tolerance and physical dependence: do they play a role in alcohol and drug self-administration? In Y. Israel, F. Glaser, H. Kalant, R.E. Popham & W. Schmidt (Eds), *Research Advances in Alcohol and Drug Problems*, Vol. 6. New York: Plenum Press.

Childress, A.R., McLellan, A.T. & O'Brien, C.P. (1986). Conditioned responses in a methadone population: a comparison of laboratory clinic, and natural settings. *Journal of Substance Abuse Treatment*, **3**, 173–179.

Cloninger, C.R. (1987). Neurogenetic adaptive mechanisms in alcoholism. *Science*, **236**, 410–416.

Cooney, N.L., Baker, L.H., Pomerleau, O.F. & Josephy, B. (1984). Salivation to drinking cues in alcohol abusers: Toward the validation of a physiological measure of craving. *Addictive Behaviors*, **9**, 91–94.

Cooney, N.L., Gillespie, R.A., Baker, L.H. & Kaplan, R.F. (1987). Cognitive changes after alcohol cue exposure. *Journal of Consulting and Clinical Psychology*, **55**, 150–155.

Corty, E., O'Brien, C.P. & Mann, S. (1988). Reactivity to alcohol stimuli in alcoholics: is there a role for temptation? *Drug and Alcohol Dependence*, **21**, 29–36.

Cotton, N.S. (1979). The familial incidence of alcoholism: a review. *Journal of Studies on Alcohol*, **40**, 89–116.

Dolinsky, Z.S., Morse, D.E., Kaplan, R.F., Meyer, R.E., Corry, D. & Pomerleau, O.F. (1987). Neuroendocrine, psychophysiological and subjective reactivity to an alcohol placebo in male alcoholic patients. *Alcoholism: Clinical and Experimental Research*, **11**, 296–300.

Drummond, D.C., Cooper, T. & Glautier, S.P. (1990). Conditioned learning in alcohol dependence: implications for cue exposure treatment. *British Journal of Addiction*, **85**, 725–743.

Ehrman, R.N., Robbins, S.J., Childress, A.R. & O'Brien, C.P. (1992). Conditioned responses to cocaine-related stimuli in cocaine abuse patients. *Psychopharmacology*, **107**, 523–529.

Eysenck, H.J. (1967). *The Biological Basis of Personality*. Springfield, IL: Charles C. Thomas.

Eysenck, S.B.G., Pearson, P.R., Easting, G. & Allsopp, J.F. (1985). Age norms for impulsiveness, venturesomeness and empathy in adults. *Personality and Individual Differences*, **6**, 613–619.

Gossop, M.R. & Eysenck, S.B.J. (1980). A further investigation into the personality of drug addicts in treatment. *British Journal of Addiction*, **75**, 305–311.

Gray, J.A. (1970). The psychophysiological basis of introversion–extraversion. *Behaviour Research and Therapy*, **8**, 249–266.

Gray, J.A. (1975). *Elements of a Two-Process Theory of Learning*. London: Academic Press.

Greeley, J., Swift, W. & Heather, N. (1992). Depressed affect as a predictor of increased desire for alcohol in current drinkers of alcohol. *British Journal of Addiction*, **87**, 1005–1012.

Greeley, J.D., Swift, W. & Heather, N. (1993). To drink or not to drink? Assessing conflicting desires in dependent drinkers in treatment. *Drug and Alcohol Dependence*, **32**, 169–179.

Greeley, J.D., Swift, W. Prescott, J. & Heather, N. (1993). Reactivity to alcohol-related cues in heavy and light drinkers. *Journal of Studies on Alcohol*, **54**, 359–368.

Heather, N. & Greeley, J. (1990). Cue exposure in the treatment of drug dependence: the potential of a new method for preventing relapse. *Drug and Alcohol Review*, **9**, 155–168.

Hodgson, R., Rankin, H. & Stockwell, T. (1979). Alcohol dependence and the priming effect. *Behaviour Research and Therapy*, **17**, 379–387.

Holland, P.C. (1983). Occasion-setting in Pavlovian feature positive discrimination. In M.L. Commons, R.J. Herrnstein & A.R. Wagner (Eds), *Quantitative Analyses of Behaviour: Discrimination Processes*, Vol. 4, pp. 183–206. New York: Ballinger.

Kaplan, R.F., Meyer, R. & Stroebel, C.F. (1983). Alcohol dependence and responsivity to an ethanol stimulus as predictors of alcohol consumption. *British Journal of Addiction*, **78**, 259–267.

Kaplan, R.F., Cooney, N.L., Baker, L.H., Gillespie, R.A., Meyer, R.E. & Pomerleau, O.F. (1985). Reactivity to alcohol-related cues: physiological and subjective responses in alcoholics and nonproblem drinkers. *Journal of Studies on Alcohol*, **46**, 267–272.

Lipscomb, T.R. & Nathan, P.E. (1980). Blood alcohol level discrimination: the effects of family history of alcoholism, drinking pattern, and tolerance. *Archives of General Psychiatry*, **37**, 571–576.

Litt, M.D., Cooney, N.L., Kadden, R.M. & Gaupp, L. (1990). Reactivity to alcohol cues and induced moods in alcoholics. *Addictive Behaviors*, **15**, 137–146.

Ludwig, A.M., Wikler, A. & Stark, L.H. (1974). The first drink: psychobiological aspects of craving. *Archives of General Psychiatry*, **30**, 539–547.

Marlatt, G.A. & Gordon, J.R. (Eds) (1985). *Relapse Prevention: Maintenance Strategies in the Treatment of Addictive Behaviors*. New York: Guilford Press.

McCusker, C.G. & Brown, K. (1991). The cue-responsivity phenomenon in dependent drinkers: "personality" vulnerability and anxiety as intervening variables. *British Journal of Addiction*, **86**, 905–912.

Monti, P.M., Binkoff, J.A., Zwick, W.R., Abrams, D.B., Nirenberg, T.D. & Liepman, M.R. (1987). Reactivity of alcoholics and nonalcoholics to drinking cues. *Journal of Abnormal Psychology*, **96**, 122–126.

Monti, P.M., Rohsenow, D.J., Rubonis, A.V., Niaura, R.S., Sirota, A.D., Colby, S.M. & Abrams, D.B. (1993a). Alcohol cue reactivity: effects of detoxification and extended exposure. *Journal of Studies on Alcohol*, **54**, 235–245.

Monti, P.M., Rohsenow, D.J., Rubonis, A.V., Niaura, R.S., Sirota, A.D., Colby, S.M., Goddard, P. & Abrams, D.B. (1993b). Cue exposure with coping skills treatment for male alcoholics: a preliminary investigation. *Journal of Consulting and Clinical Psychology*, **61**, 1011–1019.

Newlin, D.B. (1985). Offspring of alcoholics have enhanced antagonistic placebo response. *Journal of Studies on Alcohol*, **46**, 490–494.

Newlin, D.B. (1986). Conditioned compensatory response to alcohol placebo in humans. *Psychopharmacology*, **88**, 247–251.

Niaura, R., Abrams, D., DeMuth, B., Pinto, R. & Monti, P. (1989). Responses to smoking-related stimuli and early relapse to smoking. *Addictive Behaviors*, **14**, 419–428.

Payne, T.J., Schare, M.L., Levis, D.J. & Colletti, G. (1991). Exposure to smoking-relevant cues: effects on desire to smoke and topographical components of smoking behavior. *Addictive Behaviors*, **16**, 476–479.

Pomerleau, O.F., Fertig, J., Baker, L. & Cooney, N. (1983). Reactivity to alcohol cues in alcoholics and non-alcoholics: implications for a stimulus control analysis of drinking. *Addictive Behaviors*, **8**, 1–10.

Powell, J., Bradley, B. & Gray, J. (1992). Classical conditioning and cognitive determinants of subjective craving for opiates: an investigation of their relative contributions. *British Journal of Addiction*, **87**, 1133–1144.

Powell, J., Gray, J.A., Bradley, B.P., Kasvikis, Y., Strang, J., Barratt, L. & Marks, I. (1990). The effects of exposure to drug-related cues in detoxified opiate addicts: a theoretical review and some new data. *Addictive Behaviors*, **15**, 339–354.

Rankin, H., Stockwell, T. & Hodgson, R. (1982). Personality and alcohol dependence. *Personality and Individual Differences*, **3**, 145–151.

Rohsenow, D.J., Monti, P.M., Abrams, D.B., Rubonis, A.V., Niaura, R.S., Sirota, A.D. & Colby, S.M. (1992). Cue elicited urge to drink and salivation in alcoholics: relationship to individual differences. *Advances in Behaviour Research and Therapy*, **14**, 195–210.

Schuckit, M.A. (1980). Self-rating of alcohol intoxication by young men with and without family histories of alcoholism. *Journal of Studies on Alcohol*, **41**, 242–249.

Schuckit, M.A, (1984). Subjective responses to alcohol in sons of alcoholics and control subjects. *Archives of General Psychiatry*, **41**, 879–884.

Sherman, J.E., Zinser, M.C., Sideroff, S.I. & Baker, T.B. (1989). Subjective dimensions of heroin urges: influence of heroin-related and affectively negative stimuli. *Addictive Behaviors*, **14**, 611–623.

Siegel, S. (1983). Classical conditioning, drug tolerance and drug dependence. In R.G. Smart, F.B. Glaser, Y. Israel, H. Kalant, R.E. Popham & W. Schmidt (Eds), *Research Advances in Alcohol and Drug Problems*, Vol. 7, pp. 207–246. New York: Plenum Press.

Skinner, H.A. & Allen, B.A. (1982). Alcohol dependence syndrome: measurement and validation. *Journal of Abnormal Psychology*, **91**, 199–201.

Stewart, J., de Wit, H. & Eikelboom, R. (1984). Role of unconditioned and conditioned drug effects in the self-administration of opiates and stimulants. *Psychological Review*, **91**, 251–268.

Stockwell, T.R., Hodgson, R.J., Edwards, G., Taylor, C. & Rankin, H. (1979). The development of a questionnaire to measure severity of alcohol dependence. *British Journal of Addiction*, **74**, 89–95.

Tarter, R.E., Alterman, A.I. & Edwards, K.L. (1985). Vulnerability to alcoholism in men: a behavior-genetic perspective. *Journal of Studies on Alcohol*, **46**, 329–356.

Walitzer, K.S. & Sher, K.J. (1990). Alcohol cue reactivity and ad lib drinking in young men at risk for alcoholism. *Addictive Behaviors*, **15**, 29–46.

White, J.M. & Staiger, P.K. (1991). Response to alcohol cues as a function of consumption level. *Drug and Alcohol Dependence*, **27**, 191–195.

Wikler, A. (1965). Conditioning factors in opiate addiction and relapse. In D.M. Wilner & G.G. Kassebaum (Eds), *Narcotics*. New York: McGraw-Hill.

Wise, R.A. (1988). The neurobiology of craving: implications for the understanding and treatment of addiction. *Journal of Abnormal Psychology*, **97**, 118–132.

CHAPTER 6 The role of interoceptive cues for drug delivery in conditioning models of drug dependence

Janet Greeley and Colin Ryan**

INTEROCEPTIVE AND EXTEROCEPTIVE CUES

Considerable evidence exists that otherwise neutral environmental cues can come to evoke drug-related responses via the processes of classical conditioning. Distal, exteroceptive cues can only affect behaviour, of course, to the extent that the energies they emit impinge on the organism via its sensory system, to the extent that they come to be represented internally, to the extent that they percipitate interoceptive changes in state (the proximal conditioned stimulus—CS). Both distal and proximal cues are essentially symbolic in nature, triggering drug-related conditioned responses (CRs). The classical conditioning model suggests that this symbolic connection is established by repeated pairing of drug-predicated activity/experience (the unconditioned stimulus—US) and otherwise neutral features of the environment.

There is an emerging view that, just as drug-related effects can become linked to extra-organismic environmental cues, they can also link to internal states of the organism, which may or may not be accessible to introspection (e.g. mood states, withdrawal, or priming doses of the drug). Like exteroceptive or environmental cues, interoceptive cues come to elicit conditional drug-related responses. These intra-organismic cues may have an identifiable environmental trigger (e.g. pressure of work causing stress or tension which becomes a CS for, say, withdrawal-like symptoms) or may be spontaneously generated—that is, truly endogenous in origin. Identifying the environmental trigger for internal states

*James Cook University of North Queensland, Australia.

Addictive Behaviour: Cue Exposure Theory and Practice.
Edited by D.C. Drummond, S.T. Tiffany, S. Glautier and B. Remington.

(conditioned cues) is sometimes difficult and, in any event, seldom attempted. Likewise, precise specification of the internal state itself can be a hoary problem. As we will see, verifying that a priming dose of alcohol has produced a discriminable effect or that a mood-induction technique was successful is not a simple task.

COSTS AND BENIFITS OF INTEROCEPTIVE CUES

Although the notion of interoceptive cues as CSs is not new (see Bykov, 1957; Razran, 1961), its more recent reaffirmation and extension (e.g. Ader & Cohen, 1982; Solomon & Corbit, 1974) has important implications for the scope and content of conditioning theories of craving, dependence and relapse. It promises a less mechanistic theory of greater scope and generality, reflecting the fact that internal states may determine and shape human behaviour, that we are not simply environment-driven. These states, such as the early discriminative effects of drug delivery or signs of physical withdrawal, will be paired more immediately and reliably with the unconditioned reinforcing effects of the drug than most external cues (e.g. specific environments, events or individuals). In the same way, all drinkers take a first drink before proceeding with a second, third and so on.

While interoceptive cues promise a richer, more complex and more ver-idical account of drug-related behaviour, they offer a number of challenges. First, it is not enough to simply posit intra-organismic cues. They are hypothetical constructs not observable objects or events and should, accordingly, be rigorously validated using conventional methods and standards of construct validation. Secondly, one needs to resist the temp-tation to resort to unspecified or imprecise internal cues when no immediately obvious environmental CS presents itself—to resist expla-nation by "arm waving". Thirdly, explanation in terms of well-defined and assiduously validated interoceptive cues does not absolve one from the requirement to explicate the way in which the Pavlovian model applies—to specify the precise pairings, the contingencies and the associ-ations involved. It is not enough that conditioning of an internal state be a plausible explanation. Pavlovian conditioning needs to be demon-strated in the context of rigorous experimental controls and logic (cf. Glautier, Drummond & Remington, 1994).

ENTHYMEMIC EXPLANATIONS OF CONDITIONED RESPONDING

Many explanations of cue-elicited drug-related effects are enthymemic in nature, that is, logically incomplete in the sense that one or more (usually several) of the propositions which constitute the "complete" explanation are omitted. Enthymemic explanation is common in the physical sciences where the governing principles are relatively well understood and substantially agreed. It is also an integral part of common parlance. Asked why one left a garden hurriedly, one might explain that it was "because of the savage dog" without spelling out the details (general laws, initial conditions, etc) which provide logical entailment *per se* (e.g. a savage dog is likely to bite; that bite is likely to be painful and frightening; and so on). Enthymemic explanation is, then, a variety of explanatory shorthand, convenient when knowledge is shared or agreed and may be assumed, as in the case of Kuhn's (1962) paradigmatic sciences. On the other hand, enthymemic explanations can be a way of glossing over critical issues, of explaining away rather than explaining, when no genuine intellectual consensus exists.

Classical conditioning accounts of the mechanics of drug-related effects have tended to be disconcertingly enthymemic when we, in fact, know little of the underpinning processes (Stewart, 1993). Often, when an otherwise neutral external or internal "cue" apparently evokes drug-related effects, it is assumed to be a product of classical conditioning—even when the US, and the occasions and conditions of CS–US pairing, are unknown (Ehrman et al., 1992). Too often, the conditioning processes and contingencies are not spelt out; the effects are explained away by labelling a putatively once-neutral cue the CS (e.g. Saumet & Dittmar, 1985). The problem is exacerbated when the cues are hypothetical, non-observable, interoceptive states or events.

It is usual in science to demonstrate that a model applies and to test its entailments. Proponents of classical conditioning accounts of drug-related behaviour have tended, however, to assume the Pavlovian model applies simply because some putatively neutral cue evokes drug-related responses. This is to confuse the phenomenon with its explanation. Our argument here is that, while classical conditioning accounts of drug effects are often plausible and generally consistent with a great deal of data, the model should be tested directly not assumed to be true. Freudian theory—assumed to be true by many of its disciples—"explains" a great deal without risk of contradiction, but few would maintain that it is of much scientific interest.

Proponents of classical conditioning should be clear, in their own minds at least, as to whether they have genuinely tested the model as applied (was it ever seriously at risk of disconfirmation?), or whether they have simply assimilated their data to it *post hoc*. Assimilation of data often can be trivially easy if explanation is enthymemic and the use of auxiliary assumptions is unconstrained. In this sense, the classical conditioning model leads something of a double life: it has a tight logical structure that makes it appear clearly testable *a priori*, but it is indeterminate enough *post hoc* to be compatible with any outcome. We need to test classical conditioning accounts of drug-related behaviour, rather than to simply invoke them. In the next section, we examine ways in which this issue might be addressed.

EVIDENCE FOR CONDITIONING OF INTEROCEPTIVE CUES

As we have seen, there has been a tendency to attribute addicts' responsivity to naturalistic (previously drug-neutral) cues paired with drug use to Pavlovian conditioning, rather than to check that possibility directly. Robbins & Ehrman (1992) prescribe a set of criteria which must be satisfied if such attribution is to be warranted in experimental tests of cue reactivity in dependent drug users:

1. In between groups comparisons, the responding of the dependent group must be greater than that of a non-dependent control group.
2. Comparing within groups, the dependent group must show an increased response to the drug-related stimulus but not to other neutral (non-drug) stimuli.
3. If dependent subjects do exhibit generalized over-excitability, their responding to arousing non-drug stimuli must be equivalent to that of control subjects.[1]
4. Control subjects may show increased arousal to drug cues but the difference between responding to drug cues and non-drug cues must be greater for the dependent group than the control group.

We note, however, that none of the above is necessarily evidence for conditioning *per se* and none, in and of itself, is sufficient to demonstrate it.

Much of the evidence cited to support the role of classical conditioning in drug-related responding in humans has been gathered using quasi-experimental research designs, in which putative CRs have been allegedly acquired as a function of drug-use history (see Ehrman et al., 1992). The actual conditioning history of the subjects has not been controlled by the investigator: again, the CSs and their contingencies with the US are assumed, not demonstrated.

It is possible, of course, for all four criteria outlined by Robbins & Ehrman to be met and yet for the classical conditioning model to be entirely inappropriate to the explanation of cue reactivity. At best, the criteria may provide a useful preliminary framework for data screening.

In point of fact, few studies of responsiveness to naturalistic interoceptive cues for drug delivery conducted to date have met these criteria. Robbins & Ehrman have recommended a crossover design in which the responsiveness of the dependent drug users is compared across two drugs—one which is their drug of choice and one which is not (Ehrman et al., 1992). Ideally, the drug user's responses must be specific to his/her drug of choice.

A second check on whether drug-related responses to neutral cues are classically conditioned is whether they demonstrate archetypal conditioning phenomena such as extinction and conditioned inhibition. The logic here is straightforward (but flawed): a response is classically conditioned if it exhibits the phenomena usually seen with classically conditioned responses. In strict logic, of course, behaviour could mimic classical conditioning without being itself classically conditioned, and it is as well to keep this in mind. Our argument here is for a more aggressively falsificationist approach to the underpinning Pavlovian conditioning model. When checking drug-related responses for conditioning-like attributes, appropriate controls are again vital (see Newlin et al., 1989; Robbins & Erhman, 1992).

In a good deal of the research described below, the logic and detail of the application of the conditioning model are not spelled out. Drug-related responding is simply labelled rather than explained, and little discernible effort has been made to rule out viable alternative (non-Pavlovian) explanations. Some lip service is paid to alternative theories (e.g. expectancy theory) but disappointingly little effort has been made to crystallize and test the tenets which set them apart (cf. Niaura et al., 1988).

Even within the area of infra-human animal studies, where rigorous experimental control is possible, many studies are methodologically lacking (for a discussion see Westbrook & Greeley, 1992). Investigations of the role of Pavlovian conditioning in drug tolerance have typically used external stimuli as CSs. One of several exceptions is a study by Greeley et al. (1984) in which the conditioned group were given repeated pairings of a low dose of alcohol followed by a high dose of alcohol—the CS was an internal state/property/experience of the organism not an attribute of the environment. The control group received equivalent numbers of low and high dose injections but always unpaired. When tested with the low dose only, the conditioned or paired group elicited a conditioned hyperthermic response. This group also exhibited tolerance to the high dose of alcohol only if it was preceded by the low dose. In addition to demonstrating that a low dose of alcohol could serve as a CS, extinction of the CR to the low dose was also achieved through repeated injections of the low dose no longer followed by the high dose. The study is interesting in this context, in that it critically tests a classical conditioning account predicated on interoceptive cues. To date, one failed attempt to replicate this finding with another drug (morphine) has been published (Cepeda-Benito & Tiffany, 1993).[2] Researchers in the UK have attempted drug–drug conditioning with humans using two different drugs—nicotine as the CS and alcohol as the US—with mixed results (Clements et al., 1994).

In many respects, the Greeley et al. experiment with rats was an analogue of the priming dose studies conducted with humans (e.g. Hodgson, Rankin & Stockwell, 1979). With humans, however, their subjective experiences of desire for more alcohol and their perceived ability to resist further consumption were dependent variables of as much interest as changes in physiological responding. In the next section we briefly examine various classes of interoceptive cues for drug delivery.

TYPES OF INTEROCEPTIVE CUES

Priming Doses

The most commonly manipulated, and arguably the most potent of interoceptive cues for drug delivery, is the administration of a dose of the drug itself. This is known as the "priming dose" procedure in that the ingestion of a small amount of a drug is thought to "prime" the individual for the subsequent effects of a larger amount of the drug (e.g. Stewart, de Wit & Eikelboom, 1984; Stockwell, 1991). We do not propose to address the issue as to whether these so-called priming dose effects enhance the individual's appetite for the drug through positive incentive motivational processes (Stewart, de Wit & Eikelboom, 1984), or through the elicitation of withdrawal-like symptoms which provoke a kind of acquired drive state (Wikler, 1973; Siegel, 1990). Rather, we focus on (1) whether these initial drug effects serve as conditioned or unconditioned stimuli in the elicitation of increased desire for a drug and the increased likelihood of further drug consumption, and (2) whether they provide information which feeds into the beliefs of the drinker or drug user to control or modulate their feelings and actions.

The discriminable properties of drugs, and the role these play in non-medical drug use, have been the focus of a good deal of research (e.g. Overton, 1984). In infra-human animals, reinstatement of lapsed drug taking can be initiated by giving animals a priming dose of the same or a different drug (Stewart, de Wit & Eikelboom, 1984). For ethical reasons, experiments of this class have been carried out less frequently with human subjects: a selective review follows. As might be expected, the drug-use history of the volunteers has not been controlled by the investigators, but used as a non-manipulated independent variable. We examine the priming effects of alcohol first, then review key priming studies with other drugs.

Alcohol

The priming effect in humans has been studied mainly in alcoholics and other heavy drinkers after they have consumed varying doses of alcohol or placebo drinks portrayed as containing alcohol (e.g. Funderbunk & Allen, 1977; Engle & Williams, 1972; Hodgson & Rankin, 1976; Hodgson, Rankin & Stockwell, 1979; Marlatt, Demming & Reid, 1973; Merry, 1966; Rankin, Hodgson & Stockwell, 1983). Since these priming studies have been reviewed recently by Stockwell (1991), we address them here only to the extent that they are germane to the key point we wish to make: even the better research purporting to tap Pavlovian conditioning-mediated drug-related effects is problematical in many respects. For instance, while many studies purport to show a priming dose serving as CS, their designs do not permit such an unequivocal interpretation.

For example, Hodgson, Rankin & Stockwell (1979) showed that when severely dependent hospitalized alcoholics were given a high priming dose of vodka (150 ml) in the morning, 3 hours later they drank a first drink of vodka faster than when they had been given a low (15 ml) or no priming dose. It might be argued that the operative cue here is a declining blood alcohol concentration which might precipitate with-drawal-like symptoms in severely dependent drinkers. Moderately dependent alcoholics, however, showed the opposite effect, drinking their first drink more rapidly in the no priming dose condition. Irrespective of the size of the priming dose, severely dependent alcoholics reported a greater desire for more alcohol, and drank more during the afternoon drinking test than did the moderately dependent ones. Subjects were fully aware of the contents of the drinks they were given. The potential "placebo effects" (i.e. effects produced by the belief one has consumed a drug rather than the actual pharmacological effect of the drug itself) of alcohol were not addressed. There is no compelling evidence, then, that classical conditioning is implicated. Indeed, the failure of the moderately dependent group to respond to a priming dose speaks against a conditioning explanation, given that others have shown a priming effect in non-dependent social drinkers who presumably would have had less opportunity to form an association between low and higher doses of alcohol than would a group of moderately dependent drinkers (e.g. de Wit & Chutuape, 1993). de Wit & Chutuape argue that the priming effect they observed was due to the unconditioned pharmacological effect of alcohol rather than a conditioned response.

In a study by Laberg & Ellersten (1987), severely dependent inpatient alcoholics were given either soft drink or a priming dose of alcohol. They were then presented with either visual and olfactory cues for their preferred alcoholic beverage or a soft drink. Only those subjects given an alcohol priming dose showed increased desire for more alcohol and increased autonomic arousal. These effects were greater in the subjects subsequently exposed to external alcohol cues. After repeated exposure to these stimuli over 6 days, there was a decline in autonomic arousal and craving shown by the groups exposed to alcohol cues. These results were presented as evidence for a learning model of drug-related responding which declined as a result of extinction (repeated unreinforced presentations of the CS). Although alcoholics responded differently to alcohol and neutral cue conditions initially, this can, in part, be explained by the pharmacological effects of alcohol ingestion. The enhancement of this responding when actual alcohol was presented after the priming dose may have been due to a perceived continued possibility of further consumption rather than a CR to the sight and smell of alcohol. Likewise, the decline in responding over repeated cue exposures may have been due to the realization by subjects that further consumption was not possible. Alternatively, it is equally likely that other processes such as re-evaluation of the value of drinking, acquisition of distraction skills, or habituation to the exposure procedure by the subjects could also have occurred during these sessions.

Early studies on the priming effect of alcohol (Merry, 1966; Engle & Williams, 1972) emphasized the "loss of control" phenomenon described in the disease model of alcoholism (Jellinek, 1960). According to this view, one drink was believed to set off a chain reaction in the alcoholic such that he/she lost the ability to control the quantity of alcohol consumed. The "uncontrollable craving" experienced by the alcoholic after a single drink was, in these terms, an unconditioned response (UR) to alcohol due to an allergic or hypersensitive reaction. Merry (1966) found that inpatient alcoholics reported no more craving after consuming 1 fluid ounce (30 ml) of vodka disguised as a vitamin mixture than after drinking a non-alcoholic mixture. When the dose was increased to 2 ounces (60 ml) of vodka, however, virtually all alcoholics reported increased craving. It should be noted that the test with the higher dose of vodka occurred after repeated tests with the lower dose (seven tests) and the non-alcoholic mixture (eight tests). The effects of repeated measurement of craving and the passage of time in treatment may well have influenced the outcome. Furthermore, because we are not told what the levels of craving reported were, when they occurred, and if they tended to be reported more by some subjects than others, we are unable to draw any firm conclusions from this study other than that the interoceptive effect of a one ounce (30 ml) dose of vodka was not a particularly effective precipitant of craving (see also Engle & Williams, 1972).

When considering the role of priming doses as potential CSs or USs for increased craving or further consumption, it is vital to keep in mind the role of expectancies regarding the effects of alcohol. Thus, where possible, the effects of subjects' expectations about the effects of alcohol need to be controlled. One method for so doing is by using a "balanced placebo design" (Rohsenow & Marlatt, 1981). In these experiments the actual and perceived consumption of alcohol and a pharmacologically inactive substance are manipulated in an effort to disentangle the psychological and pharmacological factors involved in the observed effects of the alcohol. The study of Marlatt, Demming & Reid (1973) is often cited as a classic example of this genre. Alcoholics and a control group of social drinkers were tested under one of four experimental conditions: one group was told they were to receive alcohol and were given alcohol; another was told they would receive alcohol and were given soft drink; a third group was told they would be given soft drink and were given soft drink; while the fourth group were told they would be given soft drink and were actually given alcohol. The ruse for the study was a taste test of a new beverage which was presented either as vodka or tonic. The priming drink consisted of 2 ounces of each of the three beverages which the subjects were to evaluate in the "taste test". Thirty minutes later they were asked to compare the three beverages. They were told they could consume as much of each beverage as they liked in order to make their judgements. The experimenters unobtrusively measured the amount of each beverage drunk and used this as an index of the subjects' disposition to drink. Both groups drank more during the "taste test" when they believed that they were consuming alcohol.

As Stockwell (1991) pointed out, it is as likely that the subjects would have drunk more in the "told alcohol" condition even if they had not been given priming drinks beforehand. Because the expectations were the same for the priming manipulation and the test, it is impossible— given this design—to determine the impact of the so-called "priming dose condition". The effect of simply being asked to rate weak drinks of vodka could have as readily increased consumption compared with being asked to rate soft drinks (but see Stockwell et al., 1982; Laberg, 1986). A better comparison would have been to have all subjects rate drinks containing vodka in the "taste test". Then the expectation of receiving vodka on test would not be confounded with the pre-taste test conditions.

Walitzer & Sher (1990) conducted a study with non-alcoholic men, some of whom were deemed at risk of developing drinking problems because of a positive family history of alcoholism. In one study they were given a priming dose of alcohol in the form of their preferred beer before being presented with visual cues for beer or soda water. Both groups showed differential responding to alcohol versus non-alcohol beverage cues. These groups also showed different salivation responses after drinking placebo beer versus real beer. However, the order of presentation of the two conditions was not counterbalanced. Thus, the observed differences in responding may have been due to the timing of beverage presentations rather than some conditioned or unconditioned effect of the beverages themselves. Differences between the groups based on risk status were equivocal.

Other drugs

Studies of the priming effects of drugs other than alcohol in humans are rare. In one study, cocaine abusers were given an intravenous injection of cocaine or saline in a double-blind control procedure. They reported increased craving and wanting for cocaine 15 minutes after the intravenous injection of cocaine but not after saline (Jaffe et al., 1989). This effect was attenuated by the prior administration of the dopaminergic agonist, bromocriptine.

A search of the literature revealed no studies which specifically manipulated priming doses of nicotine as interoceptive cues for cigarette smoking. In most studies in which nicotine has been administered to smokers, it has been in a form other than cigarette smoke (e.g. nicotine gum, nasal spray, or patch) in an attempt to reduce craving and other withdrawal symptoms while avoiding the negative health effects of inhaling smoke. However, an intriguing study by Rose and colleagues suggests that sensory aspects of smoking such as the "taste" and irritant scratch in the throat produced by cigarette smoke may serve as cues or CSs for the reinforcing effects of nicotine. By partially anaesthetizing upper and lower regions of the respiratory tract they were able to alter the reported craving and desirability ratings for smoking a cigarette. If, as Rose et al. (1984) suggest, "sensory cues are important factors in smoking satisfaction" (p. 211), then manipulation of these interoceptive effects of smoking may be useful in modifying smokers' motivation to smoke.

Physiological States

In addition to the role of the interoceptive effects of the drug itself as a cue for drug delivery, internal physiological states have also been cited as common precursors to drug taking, hence candidate CSs. One such state is physiological withdrawal. Once neuroadaptation to a drug has taken place, absence of—or reduction in—the level of the drug results in the appearance of withdrawal symptoms. This disturbance can be alleviated by intake of more drug. Indeed, early theories claimed that the addict's need to relieve withdrawal was what motivated the development and maintenance of drug dependence (Lindesmith, 1968). But the occurrence of withdrawal symptoms does not necessarily lead to drug consumption (e.g. Mello, 1972). Therefore, the occurrence of drug withdrawal is not a sufficient condition to produce drug intake.

Withdrawal symptoms are unconditionally elicited by drug abstinence in individuals who are physically dependent. If the individual experiences relief from withdrawal after taking more drug then an instrumental contingency has occurred in which this behaviour becomes negatively reinforced. Of particular interest to a conditioning model of drug dependence is whether conditionally elicited withdrawal symptoms can serve as a discriminative stimulus (S^D) for drug taking. Discriminative stimuli are ones which specify when a particular action/reinforcement relationship is in operation (e.g. when the red light is on pressing the bar leads to food delivery) (Dickinson, 1980). Discriminative stimuli of this type differ from CSs in that they influence goal-directed behaviour. CSs, through Pavlovian or classical conditioning, elicit responding irrespective of its relationship to a goal. Thus, a CS paired with drug effects or drug withdrawal may elicit conditioned withdrawal symptoms. These symptoms may, in turn, serve as an S^D or an occasion setter for drug taking. Alternatively, the presence of the withdrawal state may increase the incentive value of the drug and in so doing motivate drug use. Any of these conditioned relationships could be operating but little or no effort has been made empirically to test these divergent accounts of apparent cue-elicited withdrawal signs (see Tiffany, Chapter 3).

Research has shown that by pairing environmental cues with the administration of naloxone to opiate-addicted individuals, these cues acquired the capacity to elicit withdrawal-like symptoms in the absence of naloxone (O'Brien et al., 1976; 1977). Repeated injections of saline or hydromorphone in detoxified addicts stabilized on the long-acting opiate antagonist naltrexone, also came to precipitate withdrawal signs (O'Brien et al., 1980). Self-injections administered early in treatment initially elicited positive, drug-like sensations but, as non-reinforced (i.e. effects

blocked by naltrexone) self-injections of hydromorphone and saline continued, the responses elicited were negative and withdrawal-like in nature. These studies revealed the tendency for opiate addicts to report
drug-related responses when exposed to drug injection rituals and paraphernalia or to neutral cues which had been paired with induced withdrawal states. In addition, the dissipation in responding over repeated
exposures to drug-related stimuli could be interpreted as evidence for
extinction of conditioned responding. Studies with alcoholics demonstrate that exposure to supposed cues for alcohol intake can elicit reports
of withdrawal-like symptoms (e.g. Staiger & White, 1991).

Although there are numerous anecdotal reports of elicitation of withdrawal-like states in detoxified addicts when in the presence of drug-
related stimuli, there is little compelling experimental evidence that these
are CRs (Robbins & Ehrman, 1992). While there is a nominal mapping of
these phenomena to the classical conditioning paradigm, the appropriate
control procedures were generally not employed or the sample sizes
tested were inadequate to conduct reliable statistical tests.

Moods

Another internal or interoceptive state which has been reported by drug
users to motivate drug use is changing moods (e.g. Farber, Khavari &
Douglass, 1980). Negative mood states are more commonly reported as
precipitants of drug use than are positive moods (see also Marlatt &
Gordon, 1985, p. 39; Rees & Heather, Chapter 5). In experimental studies,
mood may be induced hypnotically or manipulated by experimenter-
guided imagery.

Hypnotically induced mood states

Few experimental studies to date have attempted to manipulate mood
as a cue for drug use. In one of these studies, Litt et al. (1990) used
hypnotic suggestion to induce negative or neutral mood states in inpatient dependent drinkers. During each induced mood subjects were presented with either their preferred alcoholic beverage or seltzer water to
look at and smell. Only during induction of the negative mood state did
subjects report increased desire for alcohol when alcohol cues were present and in some subjects the negative mood state alone was sufficient
to elicit desire for alcohol. It should be noted that this study did not
employ a non-dependent control group and the role of demand characteristics in the mood induction procedure was, in our view, a serious
threat to the validity of the results.

Childress et al. (1989) employed a similar procedure with opiate addicts and compared four different mood states for their ability to elicit conditioned drug craving. They found that depression was effective on its own as an initiator of craving and signs of withdrawal. Anxiety and anger also tended to increase craving but this effect was statistically significant only when combined with exposure to the paraphernalia and procedures of the drug-use ritual. Euphoria also enhanced the craving elicited by exposure to the drug-use ritual but was ineffective on its own. Like Litt et al. (1990), these researchers did not use a non-dependent control group and did not attempt to account for the possible effects of demand characteristics. Childress et al. also noted that nine out of the ten subjects tested had been diagnosed with affective disorders in the past. This may well have influenced their susceptibility to mood changes as an inducing stimulus for drug craving. Drug use may have been an attempt to "self-medicate" negative mood states.

Imagery-induced mood states

Tiffany & Drobes (1990) have attempted to test the effects of mood on smoking urges by manipulating the affective content of imagery scripts. They used five types of script presenting positive and negative affect imagery with and without smoking urge imagery and a neutral affect script containing no smoking imagery. Unlike the studies using hypnotically induced mood, Tiffany & Drobes found that the strongest urges to smoke were elicited by affective scripts containing descriptions of smoking urges. The next most effective elicitors of reported urge to smoke were negative affect scripts without smoking urge descriptors, followed by positive affect scripts. Scripts with neutral affective content were the least effective. Although, in this study, Tiffany & Drobes did not measure changes in mood as a function of the scripts presented to subjects, they cited evidence from another study in which these same scripts evoked mood changes in the predicted direction (Maude-Griffin & Tiffany, 1994). Tiffany & Drobes countered the argument that demand characteristics could account for the observed urge ratings by pointing out the correspondence between these ratings and other smoking-related variables such as carbon monoxide level, negative affect and addiction measures. Furthermore, Tiffany & Hakenewerth (1991) showed that, when presented with these same scripts, smokers elicited different levels of autonomic arousal which, they argued, would be less likely to be affected by demand characteristics. However, in that study the self-reported urge ratings did not correspond well with the observed changes in heart rate and skin conductance. So, while autonomic arousal may not easily be affected by demand characteristics, self-report ratings could be. An important point should be made here. While we suspect the influence of demand characteristics in these mood induction studies, it is highly likely they play an equivalent role in studies where external stimuli serve as cues for conditional responding, particularly those using self-report indicators of desire or craving.

Cognitions

Each human being inhabits an abstract, richly configured, cognitive world of thoughts, expectations, memories, information, and imagination. We know from personal experience that a spectrum of irrelevant cognitions can precede a drink or cigarette. Can they be considered interoceptive cues, or should they be relegated to the status of precursor or epiphenomenon? Historically, accounts of behaviour have eschewed cognitive content as a legitimate object of analysis, while cognitivists have characterized behaviourist accounts as arid and mechanistic. Over time, of course, behaviourists have been forced to posit internal states (e.g. Tolman, 1932), and contemporary theories of animal learning emphasize the role of representations and propositions in the acquisition of Pavlovian and instrumental learning (e.g. Dickinson, 1980; Pearce, 1987). Expectancy theories of Pavlovian and instrumental conditioning have supplanted simplistic S–R accounts.

A good case exists, then, for making cognitions *per se* a pivotal concern of conditioning models, allowing the possibility of cognitions as interoceptive cues. Expectancies about a drug's effects and about one's own ability to cope with different situations (i.e. efficacy expectations) are examples of cognitions which may precede and influence drug consumption (see Marlatt & Gordon, 1985). While drug taking may occur apparently automatically under certain conditions (see Tiffany, 1990), other drug-taking episodes clearly involve a series of intentional acts. It is not yet clear whether it is useful or appropriate to consider cognitions as interoceptive cues (see Tiffany, Chapter 7).

Conclusion

The notion that intra-organismic states may act as conditional cues triggering drug-related behaviours is an important extension of traditional theory with significant implications for explaining drug dependence, craving and relapse. The range of potential CSs is extended, thereby, to the conscious and unconscious world within, posing a new order of complexity and possibility. It remains crucial, however, not simply to assume the Pavlovian conditioning model applies, or to infer that it does from observation of drug-related responses triggered by ostensibly drug-irrelevant cues. Like all scientific theories, classical conditioning accounts of drug-related behaviour are almost certainly flawed and our explanations and experiments should reflect that precept. The Pavlovian model should be routinely and systematically put at risk as we explore the processes of addiction, not merely invoked *post hoc* to account for our findings. Otherwise we may find ourselves with a theory which is consistent with everything—at odds with nothing—and what looks like good scientific news will almost certainly be bad.

NOTES

1. This particular criterion is problematic in that it may be expected that dependent drug users would react with greater levels of arousal to neutral stimuli than would non-dependent control subjects. The context in which most studies of cue reactivity take place is one in which there is an expectation on the part of the subjects that they may be exposed to drug cues. The mere anticipation of such cues might be sufficient to increase arousal levels in dependent drug users.

2. As noted by Cepeda-Benito & Tiffany (1993), this study differed from the Greeley et al. (1984) study in several ways. In particular, the doses of morphine used as CSs were effective in producing analgesic effects in and of themselves. They may also have been capable of producing amnestic effects which impaired the formation of an association between the low and high doses of the drug (for a review see Gallagher, 1985).

REFERENCES

Ader, R. & Cohen, H. (1982). Behaviorally conditioned immunosuppression and murine systemic lupus erythematosis. *Science*, **215**, 1534–1536.

Bykov, K.M. (1957). *The Cerebral Cortex and the Internal Organs*. New York: Chemical Publishing.

Cepeda-Benito, A. & Tiffany, S.T. (1993). Morphine as a cue in associative tolerance to morphine's analgesic effects. *Pharmacology, Biochemistry and Behavior*, **46**, 149–152.

Childress, A.R., Ehrman, R., McLellan, A.T., MacRae, J., Natale, J. & O'Brien, C.P. (1989). Negative mood states trigger conditioned drug craving and conditioned withdrawal in opiate abuse patients. Unpublished manuscript, Philadelphia Veterans Administration Medical Centre, Philadelphia.

Clements, K., Glautier, S., Stolerman, I.P., White, J-A.W. & Taylor, C. (1994). Classical conditioning in humans: nicotine as CS and alcohol as US. Unpublished manuscript.

de Wit, H. & Chutuape, M.A. (1993). Increased ethanol choice in social drinkers following ethanol preload. *Behavioural Pharmacology*, **4**, 29–36.

Dickinson, A. (1980). *Contemporary Animal Learning Theory.* Cambridge: Cambridge University Press.

Ehrman, R.N., Robbins, S.J., Childress, A.R., McLellan, A.T. & O'Brien, C.P. (1992). Responding to drug-related stimuli in humans as a function of drug-use history. NIDA Monograph Proceedings of IDDS Symposium/EBP Meeting, The Netherlands.

Engle, K.B. & Williams, T.K. (1972). Effect of an ounce of vodka on alcoholics' desire for alcohol. *Quarterly Journal of Studies on Alcohol,* **24**, 109–121.

Farber, P.D., Khavari, K.A. & Douglass, F.M. (1980). A factor analytic study of reasons for drinking: empirical validation of positive and negative reinforcement dimensions. *Journal of Consulting and Clinical Psychology,* **48**, 780–781.

Funderbunk, F.R. & Allen, R.P. (1977). Assessing the alcoholic's disposition to drink. In M.M. Gross (Ed.), *Alcohol Intoxication and Withdrawal* Vol. IIIB, pp. 601–620. New York: Plenum Press.

Gallagher, M. (1985). Re-viewing modulation of learning and memory. In N.M. Weinberger, J.L. McGaugh & G. Lynch (Eds), *Memory Systems of the Brain: Animal and Human Cognitive Processes,* pp. 311–333. New York: Guilford Press.

Glautier, S., Drummond, C. & Remington, B. (1994). Alcohol as an unconditioned stimulus in human classical conditioning. *Psychopharmacology* **116**, 360–368.

Greeley, J.D., Le, A.D., Poulos, C.X. & Cappell, H. (1984). Alcohol is an effective cue in the conditional control of tolerance to alcohol. *Psychopharmacology,* **83**, 159–162.

Hodgson, R. & Rankin, H. (1976). Modification of excessive drinking by cue exposure. *Behaviour Research and Therapy,* **14**, 305–307.

Hodgson, R., Rankin, H. & Stockwell, T. (1979). Alcohol dependence and the priming effect. *Behaviour Research and Therapy,* **17**, 379–387.

Jaffe, J.H., Cascella, N.G., Kumor, K.M. & Sherer, M.A. (1989). Cocaine-induced cocaine craving. *Psychopharmacology,* **97**, 59–64.

Jellinek, E.M. (1960). *The Disease Concept of Alcoholism.* Highland Park, NJ: Hill House Press.

Kuhn, T.S. (1962). *The Structure of Scientific Revolutions.* Chicago, IL: University of Chicago Press.

Laberg, J.C. (1986). Alcohol and expectancy: subjective, psychophysiological and behavioural responses to alcohol stimuli in severely, moderately and non-dependent drinkers. *British Journal of Addiction,* **81**, 797–808.

Laberg, J.C. & Ellersten, B. (1987). Psychophysiological indicators of craving in alcoholics: effects of cue exposure. *British Journal of Addiction,* **82**, 1341–1348.

Lindesmith, A.R. (1968). *Addiction and Opiates.* Chicago, IL: Aldine.

Litt, M.D., Cooney, N.L., Kadden, R.M. & Gaupp, L. (1990). Reactivity to alcohol cues and induced moods in alcoholics. *Addictive Behaviors,* **15**, 137–146.

Marlatt, G.A., Demming, B. & Reid, J.B. (1973). Loss of control drinking in alcoholics: an experimental analogue. *Journal of Abnormal Psychology,* **81**, 233–241.

Marlatt, G.A. & Gordon, J.R. (Eds) (1985). *Relapse Prevention.* New York: Guilford Press.

Maude-Griffin, P.M. & Tiffany, S.T. (1994). Verbal and physiological manifestations of smoking urges produced through imagery: role of affect and smoking abstinence. Unpublished manuscript.

Mello, N.K. (1972). Behavioral studies on alcoholism. In B. Kissin and H. Begleiter (Eds), *The Biology of Alcoholism: Vol. III, Physiology and Behavior* pp. 219–291. New York: Plenum Press.

Merry, J. (1966). The "loss of control" myth. *Lancet*, 4 June, 1257–1258.

Newlin, D.B., Hotchkiss, B., Cox, W.M., Rauscher, F. & Li, T.K. (1989). Autonomic and subjective responses to alcohol stimuli with appropriate control stimuli. *Addictive Behavior*, **14**, 625–630.

Niaura, R.S., Rohsenow, D.J., Binkoff, J.A., Monti, P.M., Pedraza, M. & Abrams, D.B. (1988). Relevance of cue reactivity to understanding alcohol and smoking relapse. *Journal of Abnormal Psychology*, **97**, 133–152.

O'Brien, C.P., Greenstein, R., Ternes, J., McLellan, T. & Grabowski, J. (1980). Unreinforced self-injections: effects on rituals and outcome in heroin addicts. *Problems of Drug Dependence*, NIDA Research Monograph 27, pp. 275–281. Washington, DC: US Government Printing.

O'Brien, C.P., Testa, T., O'Brien, T.J. & Greenstein, R. (1976). Conditioning in human opiate addicts. *Pavlovian Journal of Biological Science*, **11**, 195–202.

O'Brien, C.P., Testa, T., O'Brien, T.J., Brady, J.P. & Wells, B. (1977). Conditioned narcotic withdrawal in humans. *Science*, **195**, 1000–1002.

Overton, D.A. (1984). State dependent learning and drug discrimination. In L.L. Iversen, S.D. Iversen & S.H. Snyder (Eds), *Handbook of Psychopharmacology*, pp. 59–69. New York: Plenum Press.

Pearce, J.M. (1987). *An Introduction to Animal Cognition*. East Sussex: Lawrence Erlbaum.

Rankin, H., Hodgson, R. & Stockwell, T. (1983). Cue exposure and response prevention with alcoholics: a controlled trial. *Behaviour Research and Therapy*, **21**, 435–446.

Razran, G. (1961). The observable unconscious and the inferrable conscious in current Soviet psychophysiology: interoceptive conditioning, semantic conditioning, and the orienting reflex. *Psychological Review*, **68**, 81–147.

Robbins, S.J. & Ehrman, R.N. (1992). Designing studies of drug conditioning in humans. *Psychopharmacology*, **106**, 143–153.

Rohsenow, D.J. & Marlatt, G.A. (1981). The balanced placebo design: methodological considerations. *Addictive Behaviors*, **6**, 107–122.

Rose, J.E., Zinser, M.C., Tashkin, D.P., Newcomb, R & Ertle, A. (1984). Subjective response to cigarette smoking following airway anesthetization. *Addictive Behaviors*, **9**, 211–215.

Saumet, J.L. & Dittmar, A. (1985). Heat loss and anticipatory finger vasoconstriction induced by a smoking of a single cigarette. *Physiology and Behavior*, **35**, 229–232.

Siegel, S. (1990). Classical conditioning and opiate tolerance and withdrawal. In D.J.K. Balfour (Ed.), *International Encyclopaedia of Pharmacology and Therapeutics*, pp. 59–85. New York: Pergamon Press.

Solomon, R.L. & Corbit, J.D. (1974). An opponent process theory of motivation: I. The temporal dynamics of affect. *Psychological Review*, **81**, 119–145.

Staiger, P.K. & White, J.M. (1991). Cue reactivity in alcohol abusers: stimulus specificity and extinction of the responses. *Addictive Behaviors*, **16**, 211–221.

Stewart, J. (1993). Neurobiology of conditioning to drugs of abuse. *Annals of the New York Academy of Sciences*, **654**, 335–346.

Stewart, J., de Wit, H. & Eikelboom, R. (1984). Role of unconditioned and conditioned drug effects in the self-administration of opiates and stimulants. *Psychological Review*, **91**, 251–268.

Stockwell, T. (1991). Experimental analogues of loss of control: a review of human drinking studies. In N. Heather, W.R. Miller and J. Greeley (Eds), *Self-control and the Addictive Behaviours*, pp. 180–197. Sydney: Macmillan.

Stockwell, T.R., Hodgson, R.J., Rankin, H.J. & Taylor, C. (1982). Alcohol dependence, beliefs and the priming effect. *Behaviour Research and Therapy*, **20**, 513–522.

Tiffany, S.T. (1990). A cognitive model of drug urges and drug use behavior: role of automatic and nonautomatic processes. *Psychological Review*, **97**, 147–168.

Tiffany, S.T. & Drobes, D.J. (1990). Imagery and smoking urges: the manipulation of affective content. *Addictive Behaviors*, **15**, 531–539.

Tiffany, S.T. & Hakenewerth, D.M. (1991). The production of smoking urges through an imagery manipulation: psychophysiological and verbal manifestations. *Addictive Behaviors*, **16**, 389–400.

Tolman, E.C. (1932). *Purposive Behavior in Animals and Men*. New York: Appleton Century Crofts.

Walitzer, K.S. & Sher, K.J. (1990). Alcohol cue reactivity and ad lib drinking in young men at risk for alcoholism. *Addictive Behaviors*, **15**, 29–46.

Westbrook, R.F. & Greeley, J.D. (1992). Conditioned tolerance to morphine hypoalgesia: compensatory hyperalgesia in the experimental group or conditioned hypoalgesia in the control group? *Quarterly Journal of Experimental Psychology*, **45B**, 161–187.

Wikler, A. (1973). Conditioning of successive adaptive responses to the initial effects of drugs. *Conditioned Reflex*, **8**, 193–210.

CHAPTER 7

The role of cognitive factors in reactivity to drug cues

*Stephen T. Tiffany**

The potential role of cognitive factors in the mediation of addicts' responses to drug-relevant stimuli has long been recognized in the cue reactivity literature. For example, the later theorizing of Abraham Wikler, the originator of the idea that conditioned drug effects were central to addictive disorders, invoked cognitive constructs in an attempt to explain cue-elicited drug craving. Thus, Ludwig & Wikler (1974) stated, "Within this theoretical framework, we would consider craving for alcohol, comparable to craving for narcotics, as representing the psychological or *cognitive correlate* of a "subclinical" conditioned withdrawal syndrome" (p. 114, italics added, see also Ludwig, Wikler & Stark, 1974). They also asserted that "We would regard craving, then, as a necessary but not sufficient condition for relapse or loss of control" (p. 116). Three elements of this formulation have been repeated in most subsequent cognitive accounts of cue reactivity effects. First, nearly all cognitively framed models accept the premise that at least some component of addicts' reactivity to drug-relevant stimuli represents the operation of classical conditioning. Second, the genesis and function of craving are central concerns of all cognitive approaches to cue reactivity. Finally, most cognitive theorists have adopted the assumption that craving controls ongoing drug use in the addict and is a necessary precipitant of relapse.

This chapter will present and critique four major cognitive models adopting, to some degree, conventional views on the roles of drug craving and classical conditioning in the production of cue-reactivity effects. The appraisal of each model will be based, primarily, on empirical grounds, though in some cases, the plausibility and lucidity of key postulates will also be evaluated. The review of these models will be followed by a brief

---

*Purdue University, West Lafayette, Indiana, USA

Addictive Behaviour: Cue Exposure Theory and Practice.
Edited by D.C. Drummond, S.T. Tiffany, S. Glautier and B. Remington.
© 1995 John Wiley & Sons Ltd.

consideration of data challenging the traditional supposition, embedded within each of these models, that craving is central to all drug use. Finally, an alternative approach to the role of cognitive factors in cue reactivity will be presented. This cognitive processing model does not invoke a classical conditioning interpretation of cue reactivity effects and rejects conventional assumptions regarding the function of craving in addictive behavior.

It is important to note that the invocation of cognitive concepts in the cue reactivity literature has not been restricted to explanations of drug craving or relapse. Even classical conditioning, which is presumed by many to represent the fundamental learning process responsible for basic cue reactivity phenomena, has taken on an increasingly cognitive flavor over the past two decades. For example, many models of classical conditioning now espouse the decidedly cognitive premise that the formation of an association between two stimuli depends upon the extent to which the occurrence of one stimulus provides information about the occurrence of the other (Mackintosh, 1983; Pearce & Hall, 1980; Rescorla, 1988). Moreover, there are credible models of conditioned drug tolerance, certainly a topic of immediate relevance to cue reactivity, that use cognitive constructs such as stimulus priming, working memory, and rehearsal (e.g. Baker & Tiffany, 1985; Paletta & Wagner, 1986). Although a specific consideration of these approaches to conditioning is not particularly germane to the models presented in this chapter, the fact that cognitive constructs have exerted such a strong influence in this arena suggests that, as with the rest of psychology, studies of cue reactivity will be increasingly dominated by concepts and methods derived from the cognitive sciences (Tiffany, 1991).

COGNITIVE LABELING MODELS OF CUE REACTIVITY

Several researchers have suggested that craving represents the cognitive labeling of physiological states. These states are usually described as arising from unconditioned or conditioned drug withdrawal. In essence, this approach is an extension of Schachter & Singer's (1962) cognition-arousal theory of emotion to the problem of drug craving. In that theory, an emotional state is considered to result from an interaction between physiological arousal and a cognition appropriate to the arousal. The cognition provides an emotional label that determines the quality or content of the emotional state. The intensity of the emotion is determined by the strength of the arousal. Often, the eliciting situation provides both the arousal and sufficient information for the identifying label. Later versions of this model (e.g. London & Nisbett, 1974; Ross, Rodin & Zimbardo, 1969) attempted to clarify the vague labeling hypothesis by specifying that emotional states require arousal, appropriate emotional cognitions, and an attribution that the arousal is due to an emotional source (see review by Reisenzein, 1983).

Figure 7.1 shows how this theory might be applied to drug craving. Consider the scenario in which an abstinent alcoholic experiences strong craving to drink after walking past a bar he used to frequent. The bar cues serve as conditioned stimuli that elicit conditioned withdrawal responses. These same cues also establish a cognitive state identifying the situation as a setting for drinking. This cognition allows the alcoholic to attribute his withdrawal reaction to craving, and this craving attribution produces drug use.

Although not specifically described as such, Ludwig & Wikler's (1974) perspective on craving was clearly influenced by the cognition-arousal theory of emotion.[1] They stated that conditioned withdrawal or neurophysiological arousal was a necessary precondition for craving, but that situational factors, particularly those strongly associated with previous drug use, would determine whether the addict would consciously interpret those feelings as craving. Several other researchers have subsequently expressed the view that drug craving may arise from the labeling of physiological or affective states (e.g. Cooney et al., 1984; Drummond, Cooper & Glautier, 1990; Kozlowski & Wilkinson, 1987; Sherman et al., 1989; Shiffman, 1987), but none of these researchers has provided an extensively formulated cognition-arousal theory of craving. Perhaps the most explicit depiction of craving along these lines was supplied by Melchior & Tabakoff (1984) who hypothesized that conditioned compensatory responses to alcohol cues are interpreted, via information provided by environmental stimuli, as a desire to drink. Similarly, West & Schneider (1987) proposed that craving for cigarettes emerged from the smoker's interpretation of the physiological changes caused by nicotine abstinence as a need for cigarettes.

An evaluation of the extent to which labeling processes contribute to the genesis of craving is hampered by several factors, not the least of which is the lack of a thoroughly articulated cognition-arousal model of craving. Most cognitive-labeling conceptualizations of craving are only loose approximations of Schachter & Singer's (1963) original formulation. Moreover, they do not reflect the influential revisions of the cognition-arousal model of emotion suggested by attributional theorists (e.g. London & Nisbett, 1974; Ross, Rodin & Zimbardo, 1969). Given the absence of a formally developed cognition-arousal model of craving, it should not be surprising that there are no published studies directly testing any

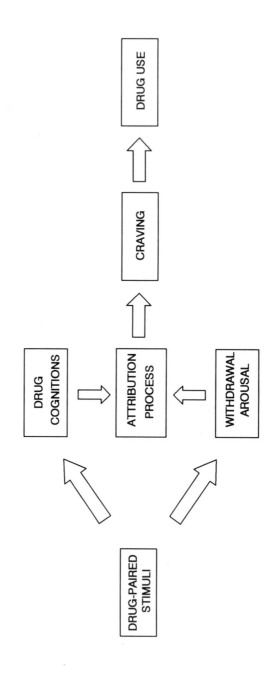

Figure 7.1 Cognitive labeling model of cue reactivity derived from Schachter & Singer's (1962) cognition arousal theory of emotion.

predictions derived from such a model. However, there are considerable data of direct relevance to a core assumption of this type of model. Schachter & Singer's (1963) theory explicitly states that the intensity of an emotional state is determined by the magnitude of physiological activity elicited by the emotional stimulus. If this model is applied to cue-elicited craving, then the magnitude of physiological reactivity elicited by drug-relevant stimuli should be strongly related to self-reported intensity of the urge state. Results from cue reactivity studies provide little support for this prediction: correlations between cue-elicited physiological effects and cue-elicited craving are generally non-significant (Tiffany, 1988, 1990).

The cognition-arousal theory of emotion has, itself, not been well supported by the data. In an extensive review of the literature, Reisenzein (1983) concluded that there was no convincing evidence that arousal is a necessary condition for an emotional state or that emotional states arise from a labeling of otherwise unexplained arousal. The decline of the influence of the cognition-arousal theory in studies of emotion can be indexed by the fact that this theory is given, at best, only cursory coverage by major contemporary emotion theorists (e.g. Frijda, 1986; Lang, 1994; Levanthal & Tomarken, 1986; Levenson, 1992). Viable theories of emotion may provide valuable sources for suggesting new methods and concepts in the study of cognitive processes in cue reactivity, but the present empirical and conceptual status of the cognition-arousal model indicates that this particular theory may have limited heuristic value for craving research.

POSITIVE EXPECTANCY MODEL OF CUE REACTIVITY

Marlatt's (1985a, c) cognitive-behavioral model of drug relapse assigns cue-elicited craving a pivotal role in the precipitation of drug use following a period of abstinence. The characterization of cue-elicited craving in this system draws heavily from expectancy-based models of learning (see Tiffany, Chapter 3, for review of animal models of expectancy), in which the presentation of stimuli previously associated with reinforcers is presumed to elicit reinforcer-specific expectancies. These expectancies are hypothesized to have both informational as well as motivational or incentive components. For example, presentation of drug-paired stimuli to an addict should generate an expectation or anticipation that use of the drug will produce specific effects such as pleasure, relaxation or relief from withdrawal as well as a desire for those particular effects. Marlatt (1985c) emphasizes that the informational content of drug-related expectancies consists primarily of anticipation of positive outcomes from drug use. He describes craving as the desire to experience those positive consequences. In essence, this model associates craving with the motivational features of positive outcome expectancies. Marlatt (1985c) also draws a distinction between craving and urges, proposing that the desire for expected positive outcomes (i.e. craving) produces urges, which represent the intention to engage in drug use.

A schematic of the positive outcome expectancy model of cue reactivity is shown in Figure 7.2. To use the earlier cited example of the abstinent alcoholic walking past a bar, the bar stimuli would elicit expectancies that drinking would produce specific effects such as pleasure, relaxation or stimulation. Those same cues would elicit a desire or craving for the specific, anticipated effects of drinking, and craving would precipitate an intention (urge) to go into the bar and order a drink. Finally, the intention to drink would produce actual drinking behavior.

There are, according to Marlatt's model, several factors that will influence the extent to which the presence of drug-paired cues will eventuate in drug use. Most importantly, the addict's level of self-efficacy, or belief in his or her ability successfully to avoid drug use in the situation, will have a major impact on whether or not confrontation with drug cues will lead to relapse. High levels of efficacy are posited to protect the addict from relapse, whereas low levels make it less likely that the addict will engage in necessary coping responses to thwart use. Craving and self-efficacy are thought to be reciprocally related. High craving, because it presents a challenge to the addict's coping skills, is hypothesized to reduce self-efficacy beliefs. Low self-efficacy should exacerbate drug craving, primarily by augmenting the incentive properties of anticipated drug effects.[2]

There has been little research specifically evaluating this expectancy-mediated model of cue reactivity. Several investigations have shown that expectancies of positive outcomes from alcohol consumption tend to be significantly correlated, concurrently and prospectively, with measures of alcohol consumption (Goldman et al., 1991; Leigh, 1989). These studies were concerned with generalized, trans-situational evaluations of expected alcohol effects, and did not explore relationships between cue-specific expectancies and levels of consumption or cue reactivity effects in the presence of alcohol cues. Consequently, their results are only tangentially pertinent to an expectancy model of cue reactivity.

In an attempt to evaluate more directly the expectancy model, Powell, Bradley and Gray (1992) explored relationships between positive outcome expectancies and reactivity to opiate cues in detoxified opiate

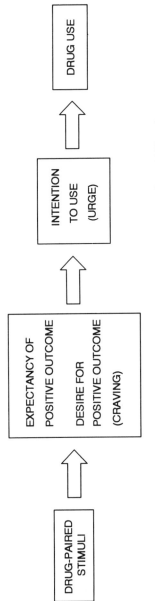

Figure 7.2 Positive expectancy model of cue reactivity (Marlatt, 1985a, c).

addicts. These researchers found that a global score from a multifactor scale of benefits of opiate use was modestly correlated with craving ratings obtained after exposure to opiate-related stimuli. Only two of the five specific expectancy scales contributing to the global scale, "emotional relief" and "lifestyle", correlated significantly with craving. The relevance of these results for Marlatt's expectancy model of cue reactivity is, for a variety of reasons, questionable. First, the assessment of expectancies focused on generalized ratings of positive outcomes collected several days prior to the attempted cue manipulation. Thus, potential relationships between cue-induced changes in expectancies and cue-specific changes in craving, which are core to evaluating the expectancy model of cue reactivity, could not be established. Furthermore, correlations were only reported between expectancy and craving ratings made following the opiate cue condition and not from the neutral condition. Therefore, the data did not address the important question of whether craving–expectancy associations were drug cue specific, as mandated by Marlatt's model, or more global, reflecting a relationship between elevated craving reports and generalized anticipation of positive outcomes from drug use.

Finally, it is unclear whether the items or the response format used in the expectancy scales developed for this study adequately represented Marlatt's (1985a, c) characterization of positive outcome expectancies. For example, the positive outcome items were heavily weighted toward anticipation of relief from dysphoric states; Marlatt emphasizes the stimulating, pleasurable effects of drugs in his depiction of positive outcome expectancies. With regard to response format, subjects were asked to rate the importance of each possible outcome in influencing his or her recent drug use. It would seem that Marlatt's (1985a, c) version of positive outcome expectancies would be better captured by a consideration of both the informational and motivational content of expectancies, that is, ratings of the extent to which a subject believed that drug use would lead to a variety of specific outcomes as well as ratings of the desirability of each outcome (e.g. Leigh, 1989).

Cooney et al. (1987) conducted a study in which changes in outcome expectancies for alcohol use were monitored in alcoholics and non-alcoholics after alcohol cue exposure. They described the outcome of their study as showing that cue exposure enhanced desire to drink and increased expectancies of positive outcomes in both subject groups. Furthermore, the alcoholic subjects exhibited a decrease in reported self-efficacy for resisting the urge to drink. Although these results appear consistent with the expectancy model of cue reactivity, close consideration of the data reveals several effects that were actually contrary to predictions of this model. Expectancies were assessed in this study via two instruments: a global rating of the pleasantness of the taste and effects of an alcoholic drink, and a 37 item scale, the Alcohol Effects Questionnaire (AEQ; Southwick et al., 1981), that yielded scores on three expectancy dimensions. Scores from the global ratings did show elevations in positive expectancies in the alcohol cue condition relative to the neutral cue condition. In contrast, scores from the more comprehensive assessment of expectancies, the AEQ, indicated that exposure to alcohol cues produced a decrease in anticipation of stimulation and dominance, no change in anticipation of pleasurable disinhibition, and a reduction in the expected behavioral impairment induced by alcohol. Ratings of desire to drink collected during alcohol cue exposure were significantly correlated with global expectancy ratings but not with any of the AEQ scales.

The authors described the AEQ results as showing that cue exposure produced "an increase in expectations that alcohol consumption will produce quieting, calming effects and improvements in concentration, coordination, and efficiency" (p. 152). If this depiction is valid, then the absence of significant correlations between the AEQ scores and desire to drink ratings would suggest that craving is not mediated by expectancies of specific positive effects. Actually, the authors' interpretation of their results is not particularly consonant with the item content of the scales nor consistent with the interpretation of these scales offered by the authors of the AEQ (Southwick et al., 1981). The AEQ data indicated that cue exposure decreased one form of positive outcome expectations (i.e. alcohol stimulation) and one form of negative outcome expectations (i.e. behavioral impairment) but had no impact on anticipation of pleasurable effects.

On balance, the results appeared to show that a global rating of positive expectancies produced results superficially compatible with aspects of Marlatt's (1985a, b) model, whereas ratings from a detailed evaluation of expectations of specific outcomes were not supportive and, perhaps, even contrary to the predictions of the model. It is important to note that, as Marlatt's model emphasizes that craving and drug use are mediated by specific, not generalized expectations of particular drug outcomes, the overall pattern of results from this study might be viewed as inconsistent with the positive outcome expectancy model of cue reactivity. A full evaluation of the relative impact of global versus specific outcome expectancies in the generation of cue reactivity effects will require the systematic development of procedures and assessments that are sensitive to the various factors that may influence these forms of expectancies.

Marlatt's (1985c) proposed distinction between the concepts of craving, as the desire for specific positive outcomes, and urge, as the intention to use drugs, has not been subjected to extensive empirical evaluation either. One problem in testing this proposal is that it is not clear whether it was meant to represent a difference in the meaning of the terms craving and urge as used by addicts, or, more likely, advocated as a terminological convention to draw an important distinction between two hypothesized aspects of drug motivational processes. Moreover, failure to find support for either a semantic or mechanistic difference between the concepts of craving and urge may not be particularly damaging to Marlatt's theory of cue reactivity, as this proposal does not appear to be central to the expectancy formulation of the model. Factor analytic studies of craving scales provide little support for a distinction between the terms urge and craving in the verbal behavior of drug users. Cigarette, cocaine and heroin addicts use the terms urge and craving nearly synonymously when describing their desire to use drugs (Tiffany & Drobes, 1991; Tiffany et al., 1993, 1994). These same studies also show that, in addicts not attempting to remain abstinent from their drug, statements of desire to use and intention to use (including craving and urge ratings) are tightly coupled. These data suggest it may not be necessary to discriminate between the terms urge and craving when assessing verbal report of drug desire (cf. Kozlowski & Wilkinson, 1987); they do not address the more important issue of whether statements of desire and intention might dissociate in situations in which an addict is trying to remain abstinent (Tiffany, 1990).

In summary, although Marlatt's (1985a, c) expectancy-based approach to cue reactivity has not been extensively explored, the few studies that have attempted directly to address the model have not yielded compelling evidence that specific outcome expectancies are core mediators of cue reactivity effects. A full evaluation of the model may first require articulation of several aspects of the theory. For example, are there configurations of drug-related cues more prone to generate global versus specific outcome expectancies? What is the relationship between specific and global expectancies in the generation of desires for drug-use outcomes? What processes control the transformation of desire for those outcomes into intentions to use drugs, and how might self-efficacy beliefs influence those processes? A clear specification of these and other features of the model may be necessary to guide systematic investigations of the contributions of expectancies to craving, urges and drug use.

DUAL AFFECT MODEL OF CUE REACTIVITY

Baker, Morse & Sherman (1987) proposed that reactivity to drug-relevant stimuli is controlled by complex, affective processing systems that can be indexed by physiological, behavioral, and self-report measures. This dual affect model proposes that reactivity can be either appetitively based (positive affect urge systems) or withdrawal based (negative affect urge systems). Positive affect urges (Figure 7.3) are assumed to be tied closely to an appetitive motivational system directly stimulated by drug administration. Activation of this network might come about through positive affect, cues previously associated with drug use, information that drug is available, and a small dose of the drug itself. When activated, this urge network should produce urge reports, positive affect, physiological responses consistent with the stimulating effects of drugs, and drug-seeking behavior. Negative affective urges are assumed to be strongly associated with drug withdrawal. Negative affect, stimuli paired with withdrawal, information that drug is not available, aversive events, and withdrawal should activate this network. When activated, this urge system should be characterized by urge reports, negative affect, withdrawal symptoms, and drug seeking. It is hypothesized that these two urge systems are mutually inhibitory; stimulation of one network should suppress the activation of the other.

Baker, Morse & Sherman (1987) propose that urge systems are structured at a cognitive level within propositional networks (e.g. Lang, 1984) that encode information on eliciting stimuli, drug-related responses, and the meaning or interpretation of stimuli and responses. These networks will be mobilized to the extent that the prevailing cue configurations provide a sufficient match for the encoded prototypical stimulus complex. An important operating characteristic of this propositional architecture is the assumption that, as the stimulus conditions approximate the prototype, the magnitude and coherence of activated response elements within a given urge network will become greater. So, for example, induction of positive mood and presentation of drug-paired cues to an addict should produce stronger responses and stronger associations between various indices of urge responding (e.g. physiological reactions and self-reported urges) than would be elicited by either of these cues presented in isolation. One other important characteristic of this propositional organization of urges is that partial activation of urge systems should reduce the threshold for additional activation of the urge network. As an illustration, ingestion of alcohol, which would produce a partial pharmacological priming of appetitive motivational systems, should specifically enhance urge reactivity to smoking-related stimuli in cigarette smokers.

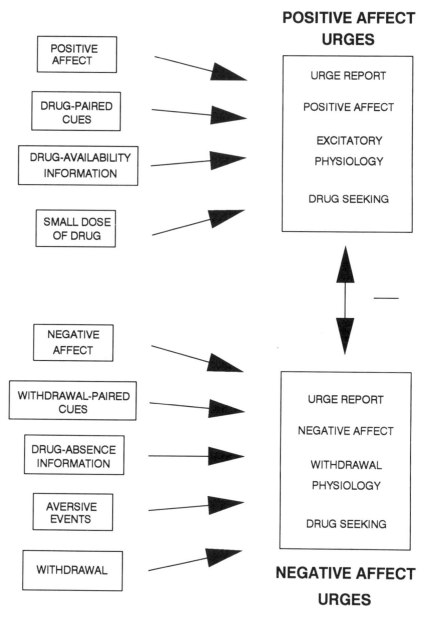

Figure 7.3 Dual affect model of cue reactivity (Baker, Morse & Sherman, 1987).

Baker, Morse & Sherman (1987) have summarized findings consistent with their characterization of the cognitive organization and motivational significance of urge reactions. The most compelling evidence concerns effects such as the facilitative impact of priming doses of drugs on self-administration (e.g. Stewart, de Wit & Eikelboom, 1984), the association of some relapses with positive mood and other appetitive stimuli (e.g. Brandon, Tiffany & Baker, 1987), the influence of signals of drug availability on urge elicitation (e.g. Meyer & Mirin, 1979), the priming of self-administration of one drug via administration of another (e.g. Henningfield, 1984), and the potential inhibitory relationships between urges associated with positive affect and urges associated with negative affect (Baker & Morse, 1985; Zinser et al., 1992). However, more recent studies designed, in part, to evaluate directly certain principal predictions of the dual affect model have yielded results discrepant with this conceptualization of cue reactivity.

The dual affect model has been challenged by the following findings.

1. An overview of the available experimental evidence shows that, in the absence of explicit drug cues, induction of positive mood generally has little or no impact on urge elicitation (Burton, Drobes & Tiffany, 1992; Litt et al., 1990; Childress et al., 1987; Elash, Tiffany & Vrana, 1994; Maude-Griffin & Tiffany, 1994; Tiffany & Drobes, 1990; see Chapter 6 for a review of the impact of mood induction on cue reactivity).
2. Urges associated with positive mood and those associated with negative mood are not necessarily mutually inhibitory. For example, factor analytic studies of multi-item craving questionnaires generally reveal that item sets reflective of anticipation of enhanced positive mood from drug use and those indicating anticipation of relief from negative mood and withdrawal are positively, not negatively, correlated (Tiffany & Drobes, 1991; Tiffany et al., 1994). Furthermore, induction of positive mood during abstinence from smoking in heavy cigarette smokers does not inhibit urge reactivity to presentations of cigarette-related stimuli (Maude-Griffin & Tiffany, 1994).
3. Partial activation of urge systems through withdrawal or pharmacological manipulations does not necessarily prime reactivity to urge-relevant stimuli. That is, abstinence from cigarettes produces general increases in urge report, but it does not selectively amplify urge reactivity to induction of negative mood or to presentations of smoking-related stimuli (Maude-Griffin & Tiffany, 1994; Drobes & Tiffany, 1994). Similarly, alcohol intoxication generally augments levels of self-reported urges to smoke but does not produce a specific amplification of urge reactivity to smoking-related stimuli (Burton & Tiffany, 1994).

4. Finally, there is little consistent evidence that the coherence of various responses to urge-eliciting stimuli becomes greater as more urge-relevant stimuli are presented to drug users (e.g. Drobes & Tiffany, 1994; Maude-Griffin & Tiffany, 1994). Actually, an examination of two major classes of cue reactions, self-reports of urges and physiological activation, reveals that in the overwhelming majority of studies there is typically little or no significant relationship between these two categories of responses (Tiffany, 1988, 1990).

Even though the validity of the affect–urge relationships posited by the dual affect model seems questionable, the conceptual and heuristic contributions of this model to cue reactivity research have been considerable. The model, in contrast to some other cognitive approaches to cue reactivity, is sufficiently formalized to allow for testing a variety of specific predictions, and it has provided a useful framework for studying mood and cue reactivity. Moreover, in presenting an explicit, rigorous account of the potential role of affect in urge processing, this model highlights the value of attending to affective variables in conceptualizing cue reactivity effects.

DYNAMIC REGULATORY MODEL OF CUE REACTIVITY

Niaura et al. (1988) integrated classical conditioning, affect regulation, and social learning concepts into a complex dynamic feedback model that attempts to describe how affective and contextual cues can precipitate relapse. This model incorporates many features of both the dual affect and expectancy-based models of drug urges in an attempt at a unified formulation of cue reactivity. A core feature of this model is the proposition that the impact of drug-relevant cues on drug use is mediated through a final pathway of self-efficacy beliefs. As depicted in Figure 7.4, contextual cues, positive affect, and negative affect can provide triggering events for a drug-use episode. These events may act singly or in concert to activate physiological responses, urges, and positive outcome expectancies. The content of these expectancies, as well as the patterning of the physiological responses, will depend, in large part, on the nature of the precipitating affect. For example, as described by Niaura et al. (1988), "If positive affect is the precipitant, outcome expectations are likely to involve anticipation of pleasurable experiences (e.g., disinhibition and increases in perceived dominance). Some physiological responses should include those indicative of anticipation of pleasure or reward" (p. 145).

These reactions to affective states and drug cues will have inhibitory

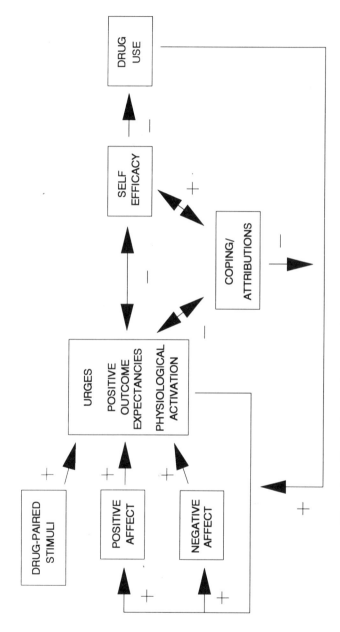

Figure 7.4 Dynamic regulatory model of cue reactivity (Niaura et al., 1988).

effects on cognitive processes that could protect the individual from drug use in this situation. Urges, physiological activation, and positive outcome expectancies should engender negative attributions that these states are uncontrollable and due to personal weakness. They will also inhibit cognitive or behavioral efforts to avoid drug use and decrease self-efficacy beliefs. The inhibitory relationships between cue reactions and these social–cognitive mediators are presumed to be bidirectional. That is, high levels of self-efficacy, attempts to cope, and positive attributions (i.e. beliefs that these states are situationally specific, unstable and controllable), will dampen reactions to affective and contextual cues. Coping efforts and attributions are assumed to interact with self-efficacy beliefs in a complementary fashion; high self-efficacy enhances coping efforts and positive attributions, low self-efficacy decreases coping and promotes negative attributions. Finally, the probability of drug use is directly determined by self-efficacy; high levels increase the likelihood that the person will avoid drug use in the situation.

The model also proposes feedback pathways that serve, in the presence of activating stimuli or actual drug use, to accentuate reactivity and further inhibit efficacy beliefs and coping efforts. For example, expectations of drug reward triggered by positive mood will, through a feedback loop, amplify that affective state, which, in turn, will elicit even greater activation of physiological reactions, urges, and positive outcome expectancies. If drug use occurs in the situation, another positive feedback pathway will be mobilized further stimulating positive and negative mood. This pathway can be inhibited to the extent that coping and positive attributions are mobilized.

The conceptualization offered by Niaura et al. (1988) is an ambitious attempt to integrate a variety of social–cognitive, conditioning, affective, and physiological concepts into a comprehensive account of the influence of drug cues and mood states on drug-use behavior. Despite the complexity of this model, inspection of the proposed sequences starting from cue exposure and culminating in drug use reveals one critical omission: there is no positive input into drug-use behavior. That is, "self-efficacy judgements are the final pathway through which all other response information gets funneled" (Niaura et al., 1988, p. 149). Self-efficacy beliefs operate to inhibit drug use in a high-risk situation; there is nothing in this model that describes how drug-use behaviors might be activated in the first place. In the absence of such an excitatory pathway, an addict in this model could, like Guthrie's (1935) characterization of Tolman's rats, be "buried in thought" and, perhaps, never at risk for relapse.[3]

The model in its current form has other features that are either conceptually implausible or incomplete from the perspective of contemporary social–cognitive approaches to drug relapse. For example, the proposed positive feedback pathway from cue reactions to mood states presents, in the terms of systems theory (DiStefano, Stubberud & Williams, 1990), an example of an unstable or, potentially, explosive system. There is no mechanism in this regulatory circuitry to prevent any low intensity mood state from invariably escalating into an intense affective reaction. The model also provides no path that can explain findings that situational or affective factors may influence the generation of coping behaviors or self-efficacy judgements, effects not necessarily dependent on the elicitation of urges, physiological activation or positive outcome expectancies (e.g. Drobes, Meier & Tiffany, 1994; Shiffman & Jarvik, 1987). Most theoreticians who invoke coping or self-efficacy as mediators of relapse recognize that these processes can be modified directly by mechanisms outside those posited in this regulatory model (e.g. Marlatt, 1985a, c; Wills & Shiffman, 1985).

In addition to these potential structural limitations, there are data that challenge some core assumptions of this model. For example, the model proposes that both positive and negative mood should function as potent cues in the elicitation of drug urges and other indices of cue reactivity. As noted above, in experimental studies of mood and urge manipulation, positive mood states are not particularly effective in inducing urges.

Data from a recent coping response study by Drobes, Meier & Tiffany (1994) also challenge other key propositions of the regulatory model of cue reactivity. These researchers had abstinent smokers who had just completed a smoking cessation treatment program vividly imagine audiotaped depictions of high-risk scenarios. At the end of the presentation of each scenario, subjects were asked to state what they would do in that situation, and they then provided ratings of their reactions to the situation. The subjects' verbal statements were coded to assess the latency, length, number, and type of coping responses generated for each situation. Follow-up data were then collected for 1 year to establish the exact number of days until the first relapse episode after treatment for each subject. In contrast to Niaura et al.'s (1988) proposal that coping responses and self-efficacy judgements should be directly related, this study revealed no significant associations between self-efficacy ratings and any measure of coping. Even more damaging for the regulatory model, both self-efficacy ratings and coping measures significantly predicted latency to first relapse, yet the contributions of coping to the prediction of relapse were independent of the relationship between self-efficacy and relapse. Thus, these data disconfirm the central proposition of the dynamic regulatory model that self-efficacy beliefs provide a common final pathway for the integration of all cue reactivity effects in the production of relapse.

EVALUATION OF COMMON ASSUMPTIONS

Over the past two decades, more than a hundred studies have shown that addicts respond to presentations of drug-relevant stimuli with increases in self-reports of urges and craving, various changes in patterns of autonomic responding, and, in some cases, increases in drug seeking or drug consumption (Baker, Morse & Sherman, 1987; Niaura et al., 1988; Rohsenow et al., 1990). Despite considerable differences among the models described above in terms of the specific cognitive processes used to explain these cue reactivity effects, they all share two fundamental assumptions. First, in common with nearly all theories of cue reactivity, these models view addicts' reactions to drug-relevant stimuli as representing, predominantly, the operation of classical conditioning. Second, these models assert that urges or craving are subjective states that represent the primary motivational processes responsible for drug use in addicts. These motivational states should be manifest through parallel changes in self-reported desire to use drugs, drug-use behavior, and, in many conceptualizations, characteristic patterns of physiological responses. A direct implication of this view is that craving is a necessary precursor to all drug-use episodes. The notion that, in addicts, craving is responsible for drug use is certainly not restricted to cognitive models of cue reactivity. This assumption has dominated the addictions field for at least a century and remains at the core of nearly all modern conceptualizations of drug addiction (Tiffany, in press).

The popularity of the idea that craving drives all drug use is surprising in view of the fact that it has scant empirical support. For example, Tiffany (1990) reviewed cue reactivity studies in which both self-reported craving and drug administration behavior were monitored. Correlations between these two measures tended to be modest, at best, and were nonsignificant in many studies (also see Kassel & Shiffman, 1992). Furthermore, there are several published cases of temporal dissociations between measures of self-reported craving and drug use. Some recent examples can be found in evaluations of the treatment efficacy of nicotine patches. This research demonstrates that decreases in smoking behavior associated with patch use may be accompanied by diminished craving report. However, in some of these studies, reductions in craving lag reductions in smoking (Abelin et al., 1989; Tønnesen et al., 1991). There are also numerous examples in which interventions reduced drug intake but had little effect on craving report (e.g. Gross & Stitzer, 1989; Nemeth-Coslett & Henningfield, 1986), or reduced self-reports of craving but had no impact on drug use (e.g. Fischman et al., 1990). Finally, relapsed addicts rarely spontaneously identify urges and cravings as immediate, major contributors to their drug relapse episodes (e.g. Chaney, Roszell & Cummings, 1982; Cummings, Gordon & Marlatt, 1980; Heather, Stallard & Tebbutt, 1991; Marlatt & Gordon, 1980; O'Connell & Martin, 1987). In fact, many addicts, if explicitly asked, will deny experiencing any urges or cravings just prior to their relapse (e.g. Baer et al., 1989).

COGNITIVE PROCESSING MODEL OF CUE REACTIVITY

Tiffany (1990) presented a cognitive processing model of cue reactivity that explicitly rejects the assumption that craving represents the central motivational process responsible for drug-use behavior. According to this theory, the mechanisms linking drug-related stimuli to drug-use behavior operate independently of the processes that control craving. The model also asserts that physiological reactions to drug-related stimuli are not necessarily classically conditioned responses, but may reflect, instead, the cognitive and behavioral demands of the drug-use situation.

The cognitive processing model draws on the strong parallels between various descriptions of automatic and non-automatic cognitive processing (e.g. Logan, 1988; Posner & Snyder, 1975; Schneider, 1985; Schneider, Dumais & Shiffrin, 1984; Shiffrin & Schneider, 1977) and key characteristics of drug use and drug urges. It is generally acknowledged by cognitive theorists that, with repeated practice, performance of cognitive or motor tasks becomes increasingly effortless, efficient, and stimulus bound, and can be carried out with little or no awareness of the component actions. This transformation of performance as a consequence of practice is assumed to represent the development of automaticity, and this mode of cognitive functioning is believed to regulate most of the daily activities of humans. This theory suggests that, as a result of a long history of practice, drug-use behavior in the addict becomes automatized. That is, like all other automatized skills, drug use becomes fast and efficient, steroryped, stimulus bound, cognitively effortless, difficult to impede, and capable of being initiated and completed without intention. These automatized skills are stored in long-term memory in the form of action schemata, which are unitized, self-sufficient memory systems containing adequate information for the initiation and coordination of complex sequences of drug-use behavior.

The proposed chain of events involved in a drug-use episode is shown on the left side of Figure 7.5. Some configuration of stimulus events activates a drug-use action schema controlling drug-use behavior. The degree to which particular stimuli elicit automatized schemata will depend on the extent to which those stimuli had been consistently associated with previous episodes of drug seeking and drug use. Encoded within these memory systems is information specifying stimulus configurations necessary for the elicitation and coordination of component actions. These might include drug-use environments (e.g. a bar room), specific drug stimuli (e.g. a bottle of alcohol, the smell of a cigarette), activation of emotional networks (e.g. anger), physical states (e.g. withdrawal), or specific drug effects. These memory structures also include information on procedures for the enactment of specific drug-use actions, coordination of actions into drug-use sequences, alternative action sequences in the event of minor obstacles to the execution of the schemata, support physiology for the metabolic demands of the action components, and generation of physiological adjustments in anticipation of drug intake.

In this model, urges and cravings are conceptualized as constellations of verbal, somatovisceral and behavioral responses supported by non-automatic cognitive processes. Non-automatic processes are believed to

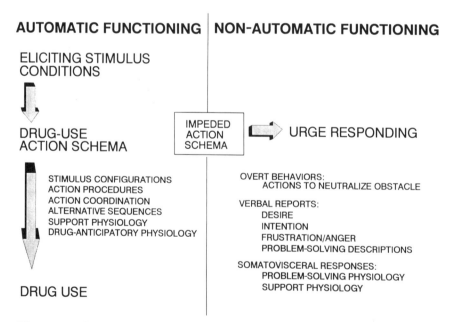

Figure 7.5   Cognitive processing model of cue reactivity (Tiffany, 1990).

be slow, dependent upon intention, flexible, cognitively effortful, and restricted by limited cognitive capacity (e.g. Shiffrin & Schneider, 1977). This mode of processing is required in situations in which automatic processes have not or cannot be invoked to produce appropriate responses. One situation requiring considerable non-automatic processing is one in which the individual is attempting to thwart or prevent the execution of an automatized sequence (Norman & Shallice, 1985; Schneider, Dumais & Shiffrin, 1984).

The model hypothesizes that non-automatic processes would be activated in parallel with drug-use action schemata either in support of the schema, as would happen when some environmental obstacle impedes or blocks an addict's attempt to use drugs, or in an effort to block the automatized sequence from going through to completion, as would occur when the addict is attempting abstinence. As an example of the former situation, what would happen if an alcoholic went to a local tavern to drink, only to discover that the establishment had been closed by the board of health? This predicament will require non-automatic cognitive processing to permit the completion of the drug-use action schema.

The right side of Figure 7.5 depicts the three broad classes of behavioral manifestations of urges that would be activated in this kind of situation. Verbal reports would include statements of craving and desire to drink, intention to drink, frustration and annoyance, and, if prompted, descriptions of problem solving engaged to surmount the obstacle to drinking. Overt behavior would consist of actions to overcome or neutralize the obstacle, e.g. running to another tavern. Physiological responses should reflect the cognitive demands of the problem situation and the metabolic demands of the overt behaviors initiated to deal with the impediment to drinking. This last proposal is predicated on well-established findings that cognitively challenging tasks (see Casper & Kantowitz, 1987, for review) and execution and even anticipation of physically demanding tasks (e.g. Elliot, 1974; Obrist et al., 1970) have pronounced effects on somatovisceral responses.

With few exceptions (e.g. Meyer, 1988; Powell, Bradley & Gray, 1992), most cue reactivity researchers have adopted uncritically the view that all physiological reactions to drug-paired stimuli are mediated primarily through classical conditioning. One important implication of the cognitive processing theory is that many of the physiological changes accompanying urge reports may represent reactions to the behavioral or cognitive demands of the situation, and are not classically conditioned drug-withdrawal or drug-appetitive effects. More generally, according to this theory, somatovisceral responses elicited by drug cue manipulations are likely to be multiply determined, perhaps reflecting elements of physiological reactions encoded within obstructed action schema as well as the behavioral and cognitive requirements of the eliciting predicament. If all, or even some, of these factors contribute to cue reactivity effects, then it would be impossible to identify a uniform physiology of drug craving. This also suggests that cue reactivity researchers might have to move beyond classical conditioning interpretations and begin evaluating their physiological data from the broader perspective offered by cognitive psychophysiology (e.g. Jennings & Coles, 1991).

The cognitive processing model provides many specific predictions about the structure of urge report and its relationship to drug use, the organization of drug-use behavior, and the role of automatic and non-automatic processes in drug relapse. The extant data on drug urges and the relationship of urges to drug use are generally compatible with this cognitive approach, but, because the model is new, few of its specific predictions have been investigated. However, the model does make several predictions about the various behavioral manifestations of urge processing that have been tested. Of particular relevance to cue reactivity research, the model hypothesizes that the operation of of non-automatic processes giving rise to urge responding should be associated with interference on concurrent tasks also requiring non-automatic processing for their successful completion. The results of several studies suggest urges may disrupt effortful cognitive processes. For example, Brandon, Tiffany & Baker (1987) found that the majority of abstinent smokers who said urges were affecting their lives stated specifically that smoking urges were disrupting their thinking or functioning. More recently, in a laboratory study of urge induction, Wetter, Brandon & Baker (1992) found that urge report was significantly associated with the number of errors made in a tracing task.

Experimental manipulations of smoking urges have produced more direct evidence of the deleterious effect of urges on cognitive processing. Drobes, Meier & Tiffany (1994) found that the incorporation of explicit urge material into coping scenarios presented to abstinent smokers increased the latency for the generation of coping responses, suggesting that urge elicitation disrupted coping. Droungas et al. (1992) reported that elicitation of smoking urges through the *in vivo* and imaginal presentation of smoking cues significantly attenuated performance on a cognitively demanding Stroop task. Recently, Sayette et al. (1994) demonstrated that alcoholics responded more slowly to tone probes presented in the presence of an alcohol beverage than in the presence of a control beverage. Finally, Cepeda-Benito & Tiffany (1994) obtained clear evidence across two studies of a disruptive effect of smoking urge elicitation on a secondary reaction time task. These diverse effects of urge elicitation on various measures of cognitive performance, which are not anticipated by the other models reviewed in this chapter, are consistent with the proposal that urges reflect the operation of effortful cognitive processes (Tiffany, 1990).

SUMMARY AND CONCLUSIONS

The models described in this chapter provide varying perspectives on the degree to which cognitive processes must be invoked to supplement or even supplant traditional conditioning theories of cue reactivity phenomena. Despite their differences, all of these models presume that interpretations based solely on classical conditioning cannot adequately predict or explain the panoply of responses elicited by manipulations of drug cues. These models also suggest that reactions to drug-paired stimuli might be manifest through changes in variables beyond the standard inventory of cue reactivity effects. That is, in addition to changes in craving, autonomic responding, and drug use, presentations of drug cues might influence attributions, outcome expectancies, self-efficacy, drug-use intentions, and performance-based indices of cognitive processing. Thus, cognitive approaches offer mechanisms and measures not envisioned by simple conditioning models of cue reactivity.

Although these cognitive models question whether classical conditioning can provide a complete explanation for cue reactivity phenomena, none challenges the value of the cue reactivity paradigm for studying addictive disorders. The relevance of this paradigm for investigating processes fundamental to addictive behavior transcends the validity of any particular cognitive or non-cognitive model of cue reactivity effects. Any comprehensive model of addiction will have to account for the complex of reactions displayed by addicts confronted with drug-relevant stimuli.

ACKNOWLEDGEMENTS

Preparation of this chapter was facilitated by a research grant (PBR 44) from the American Cancer Society. Kristine Tiffany, Antonio Cepeda-Benito, Susan Burton, Brian Carter, Celeste Elash, and Lisa Sanderson provided useful comments on drafts of this chapter. Peggy Treece helped prepare the manuscript.

NOTES

1. Schachter & Singer (1962) were cited by Ludwig & Wikler (1974) in support of an assertion that physiological states and drug effects were readily manipulable

through experimental factors. The cognition arousal theory of emotion was not cited in support of the cognitive model of craving described by Ludwig & Wikler (1974).

2. Marlatt's conceptualizations of craving have not been limited to those suggested in this synopsis of his model. In addition to the expectancy viewpoint, he also endorsed cognition arousal mechanisms of craving. For example, in the same book in which the expectancy model of craving is described, Marlatt (1985b) stated, "an urge is experienced as a response to a specific stressful situation—a state of arousal or tension that comes to be labeled as an urge or a state of craving" (p. 86). In another chapter, Marlatt (1985c) asserted, "an individual who is experiencing increased emotional arousal in a high-risk situation may misinterpret this reaction as craving for the drug rather than attributing it to the stress of the situation itself" (pp. 141–142). It is unclear whether the operation of these cognition arousal mechanisms is meant to complement or replace expectancy-based craving processes. There has been no attempt in Marlatt's writings to integrate the expectancy and cognition arousal processes into a unified model of craving.

3. Guthrie (1935) in his critique of Tolman's (1932) cognitive approach to learning stated, "In his concern with what goes on in the rat's mind, Tolman has neglected to predict what the rat will do. So far as the theory is concerned the rat is left buried in thought" (p. 143).

REFERENCES

Abelin, T., Buehler, A., Muller, P., Vesanen, K. & Imhof, P.R. (1989). Controlled trial of transdermal nicotine patch in tobacco withdrawal. *Lancet*, **1**. 7–9.

Baer, J.S., Kamark, T., Lichtenstein, E. & Ransom, C.C. (1989). Prediction of smoking relapse: analyses of temptations and transgressions after initial cessation. *Journal of Consulting and Clinical Psychology*, **57**, 623–627.

Baker, T.B. & Morse, E. (1985). The urge as affect. Paper presented at the convention of the Association for the Advancement of Behavior Therapy, Houston.

Baker, T.B. & Tiffany, S.T. (1985) Morphine tolerance as habituation. *Psychological Review*, **92**, 78–108.

Baker, T.B., Morse, E. & Sherman, J.E. (1987). The motivation to use drugs: a psychobiological analysis of urges. In P.C. Rivers (Ed.), *The Nebraska Symposium on Motivation: Alcohol Use and Abuse*, pp. 257–323. Lincoln: University of Nebraska Press.

Brandon, T.H., Tiffany, S.T. & Baker, T.B. (1987). Characterization of the process of smoking relapse. In F. Tims & C. Leukefeld (Eds), *Relapse and Recovery in Drug Abuse*, NIDA Research Monograph, No. 72, pp. 104–117. Washington, DC: US Government Printing Office.

Burton, S. & Tiffany, S.T. (1994). Impact of alcohol intoxication on reactivity to smoking-related cues. Manuscript submitted for publication.

Burton, S., Drobes, D.J. & Tiffany, S.T. (1992). The manipulation of mood and smoking urges through imagery: evaluation of facial EMG activity. Paper presented at the annual meeting of the Midwestern Psychological Association, Chicago.

Cepeda-Benito, A. & Tiffany, S.T. (1994). The use of a dual-task procedure for the assessment of cognitive effort associated with smoking urges. Manuscript submitted for publication.

Chaney, E.F., Roszell, D.K. & Cummings, C. (1982). Relapse in opiate addicts: a behavioral analysis. *Addictive Behaviors*, **7**, 291–297.

Childress, A.R., McLellan, A.T., Ehrman, R. & O'Brien, C.P. (1987). Mood states can elicit conditioned withdrawal and conditioned craving in opiate abuse patients. In L.S. Harris (Ed.), *Problems of Drug Dependence 1986*, National Institute on Drug Abuse Monograph 76, pp. 137–144. Washington, DC: US Government Printing Office.

Cooney, N.L., Baker, L.H., Pomerleau, O.F. & Josephy, B. (1984). Salivation to drinking cues in alcohol abusers: toward the validation of a physiological measure of craving. *Addictive Behaviors*, **9**, 91–94.

Cooney, N.L., Gillespie, R.A., Baker, L.H. & Kaplan, R.F. (1987). Cognitive changes after alcohol cue exposure. *Journal of Consulting and Clinical Psychology*, **55**, 150–155.

Cummings, C., Gordon, J. & Marlatt, G.A. (1980). Relapse: strategies of prevention and prediction. In W.R. Miller (Ed.), *The Addictive Behaviors*. Oxford: Pergamon Press.

DiStefano, J.J., Stubberud, A.R. & Williams, I.J. (1990). *Schaums's Outline of Theory and Problems of Feedback and Control Systems*, 2nd edn. New York: Graw-Hill.

Drobes, D.J. & Tiffany, S.T. (1994). Comparisons of smoking urges elicited through imagery and *in vivo* cue exposure. Manuscript submitted for publication.

Drobes, D.J., Meier, E.A. & Tiffany, S.T. (1994). Assessment of the effects of urges and negative affect on smokers' coping skills. *Behaviour Research and Therapy*, **32**, 165–174.

Droungas, A., Childress, A.R., Ehrman, R., Semans, M. & O'Brien, C. (1992). Effect of smoking cues on physiological reactivity, subjective report of craving and latency to smoke in smokers. Paper presented at the International Narcotics Research Conference, Keystone, Colorado.

Drummond, D.C., Cooper, T. & Glautier, S.P. (1990). Conditioned learning in alcohol dependence: implications for cue exposure treatment. *British Journal of Addiction*, **85**, 725–743.

Elash, C.A., Tiffany, S.T. & Vrana, S.R. (1995). The manipulation of smoking urges through a brief imagery procedure: self-report, psychophysiological, and startle-probe responses. *Experimental and Clinical Psychopharmacology*, in press.

Elliott, R. (1974). The motivational significance of heart rate. In P.A. Obrist, A.H. Black, J. Brener & L.V. DiCara (Eds), *Cardiovascular Psychophysiology: Current Issues in Response Mechanisms, Biofeedback and Methodology*, pp. 505–537. Chicago: Aldine.

Fijda, N.H. (1986). *The Emotions*. Cambridge: Cambridge University Press.

Fischman, M.W., Foltin, R.W., Nestadt, G. & Pearlson, G.D. (1990). Effects of desipramine maintenance on cocaine self-administration by humans. *Journal of Pharmacology and Experimental Therapeupics*, **253**, 760–770.

Goldman, M.S., Brown, S.A., Christiansen, B.A. & Smith, G.T. (1991). Alcoholism and memory: Broadening the scope of alcohol-expectancy research. *Psychological Bulletin*, **110**, 137–146.

Gross, J. & Stitzer, M.L. (1989). Nicotine replacement: ten-week effects on tobacco withdrawal symptoms. *Psychopharmacology*, **98**, 334–341.

Guthrie, E.R. (1935). *The Psychology of Learning*. New York: Harper.

Heather, N., Stallard, A. & Tebbutt, J. (1991). Importance of substance cues in relapse among heroin users: comparison of two methods of investigation. *Addictive Behaviors*, **16**, 41–49.

Henningfield, J.E. (1984). Behavioral pharmacology of cigarette smoking. In T. Thompson, P.B. Dews & J.E. Barrett (Eds), *Advances in Behavioral Pharmacology*, Vol. 4. New York: Academic Press.

Jennings, J.R. & Coles, M.G.H. (1991). *Handbook of Cognitive Psychophysiology: Central and Autonomic Nervous System Approaches*. New York: John Wiley.

Kassel, J.D. & Shiffman, S. (1992). What can hunger teach us about drug craving? A comparative analysis of the two constructs. *Advances in Behavior Research and Therapy*, **14**, 141–167.

Kozlowski, L.T. & Wilkinson, D.A. (1987). Use and misuse of the concept of craving by alcohol, tobacco, and drug researchers. *British Journal of Addiction*, **82**, 31–36.

Lang, P.J. (1984). Cognition in emotion: concept and action. In C. Izard, J. Kagan & R. Zajonc (Eds), *Emotion, Cognition and Behavior*, pp. 192–226. New York: Cambridge University Press.

Lang, P.J. (1994). The motivational organization of emotion: affect–reflex connections. In S. Van Goozen, N.E. van de Pol & J.A. Sergeant (Eds), *The emotions: Essays on Emotion Theory*. pp. 61–93. Hillsdale, NJ: Erlbaum.

Leigh, B.C. (1989). In search of the seven dwarves: issues in measurement and meaning in alcohol expectancy research. *Psychological Bulletin*, **105**, 361–373.

Levanthal, H. & Tomarken, A.J. (1986). Emotion: today's problems. *Annual Review of Psychology*, **37**, 565–610.

Levenson, R.W. (1992). Autonomic nervous system differences among emotions. *Psychological Science*, **3**, 23–27.

Litt, M.D., Cooney, N.L., Kadden, R.M. & Gaupp, L. (1990). Reactivity to alcohol cues and induced moods in alcoholics. *Addictive Behaviors*, **15**, 137–146.

Logan, G.D. (1988). Toward an instance theory of automatization. *Psychological Review*, **95**, 492–527.

London, H. & Nisbett, R.E. (1974). Elements of Schachter's cognitive theory of emotional states. In H. London and R.E. Nisbett (Eds), *Thought and Feeling*. Chicago: Aldine.

Ludwig, A.M. & Wikler, A. (1974). "Craving" and relapse to drink. *Quarterly Journal of Studies on Alcoholism*, **35**, 108–130.

Ludwig, A.M., Wikler, A. & Stark, L.H. (1974). The first drink: psychobiological aspects of craving. *Archives of General Psychiatry*, **30**, 539–547.

Mackintosh, N.J. (1983). *Conditioning and Associative Learning*. Oxford: University Press.

Marlatt, G.A. (1985a). Relapse prevention: theoretical rationale and overview of the model. In G.A. Marlatt & J.R. Gordon (Eds), *Relapse Prevention*, pp. 3–70. New York: Guilford Press.

Marlatt, G.A. (1985b). Situational determinants of relapse and skill-training interventions. In G.A. Marlatt & J.R. Gordon (Eds), *Relapse Prevention*, pp. 71–127. New York: Guilford Press.

Marlatt, G.A. (1985c). Cognitive factors in the relapse process. In G.A. Marlatt & J.R. Gordon (Eds), *Relapse Prevention*, pp. 128–200. New York: Guilford Press.

Marlatt, G.A. & Gordon, J.R. (1980). Determinants of relapse: implications for the maintenance of behavior change. In P.O. Davidson & S.M. Davidson (Eds), *Behavioral Medicine: Changing Health Lifestyles*, pp. 410–452. New York: Brunner/Mazel.

Maude-Griffin, P.M. & Tiffany, S.T. (1994). Verbal and physiological manifestations of smoking urges produced through imagery: role of affect and smoking abstinence. Manuscript submitted for publication.

Melchior, C.L. & Tabakoff, B. (1984). A conditioning model of alcohol tolerance. In M. Galanter (Ed), *Recent Developments in Alcoholism*, Vol. 2, pp. 5–16. New York: Plenum Press.

Meyer, R.E. (1988). Conditioning phenomena and the problem of relapse in opioid addicts and alcoholics. In A.B. Ray (Ed.), *Learning Factors in Substance Abuse*, pp. 161–179. Washington, DC: US Department of Health and Human Services.

Meyer, R.E. & Mirin, S.M. (1979). *The Heroin Stimulus: Implications for a Theory of Addiction*, pp. 231–247. New York: Plenum Press.

Nemeth-Coslett, R. & Henningfield, J.E. (1986). Effects of nicotine chewing gum on cigarette smoking and subjective and physiologic effects. *Clinical Pharmacology and Therapy*, **39**, 625–630.

Niaura, R.S., Rohsenow, D.J., Binkoff, J.A., Monti, P., M., Pedraza, M. & Abrams, D.B. (1988). Relevance of cue reactivity to understanding alcohol and smoking relapse. *Journal of Abnormal Psychology*, **97**, 133–152.

Norman, D.A. & Shallice, T. (1985). Attention to action: willed and automatic control of behavior. In R.J. Davidson, G.E. Schwartz & D. Shapiro (Eds), *Consciousness and Self-regulation: Vol. 4. Advances in Research and Theory*, pp. 2–18. New York: Plenum Press.

Obrist, P.A., Webb, R.A., Sutterer, J.R. & Howard, J.L. (1970). The cardia-somatic relationship: some reformulations. *Psychophysiology*, **6**, 569–587.

O'Connell, K.A. & Martin, E.J. (1987). Highly tempting situations associated with abstinence, tempory lapse, and relapse among participants in smoking cessation programs. *Journal of Consulting and Clinical Psychology*, **55**, 367–371.

Paletta, M.S. & Wagner, A.R. (1986). Development of context-specific tolerance to morphine: support for a dual-process interpretation. *Behavioral Neuroscience*, **100**, 611–623.

Pearce, J.M. & Hall, G. (1980). A model for Pavlovian conditioning: variations in the effectiveness of conditioned but not of unconditioned stimuli. *Psychological Review*, **87**, 532–552.

Posner, M.I. & Snyder, C.R.R. (1975). Attention and cognitive control. In R.L. Solso (Ed.), *Information Processing and Cognition: The Loyala Symposium*, pp. 55–85. New York: John Wiley.

Powell, J., Bradley, B. & Gray, J. (1992). Classical conditioning and cognitive determinants of subjective craving for opiates: an investigation of their relative contributions. *British Journal of Addiction*, **87**, 1133–1144.

Reisenzein, R. (1983). The Schachter theory of emotion: two decades later. *Psychological Bulletin*, **94**, 239–264.

Rescorla, R.A. (1988). Pavlovian conditioning: it's not what you think it is. *American Psychologist*, **43**, 151–160.

Rohsenow, D.J., Niaura, R.S., Childress, A.R., Abrams, D.B., and Monti, P.M. (1990). Cue reactivity in addictive behaviors: theoretical and treatment implications. *International Journal of the Addictions*, **25**, 957–993.

Ross, L., Rodin, J. & Zimbardo, P.G. (1969). Toward an attribution therapy: the reduction of fear through induced cognitive-emotional misattribution. *Journal of Personality and Social Psychology*, **12**, 279–288.

Sayette, M.A., Monti, P.M., Rohsenow, D.J., Bird-Gulliver, S., Colby, S., Sirota, A., Niaura, R.S. & Abrams, D.B. (1994). The effects of cue exposure on reaction time in alcoholics. *Journal of Studies on Alcohol*, **55**, 629–633.

Schachter, S. & Singer, J.E. (1962). Cognitive, social, and physiological determinants of emotional state. *Psychological Review*, **69**, 379–399.

Schneider, W. (1985). Toward a model of attention and the development of automatic processing. In M.E. Posner & O.S.M. Martin (Eds), *Attention and Performance XI*, pp. 475–492. Hillsdale, NJ: Lawrence Erlbaum.

Schneider, W., Dumais, S.T. & Shiffrin, R.M. (1984). Automatic and control processing and attention. In R. Parasuraman & D.R. Davies (Eds), *Varieties of Attention*, pp. 1–25. Orlando: Academic Press.

Sherman, J.E., Zinser, M.C., Sideroff, S.I. & Baker, T.B. (1989). Subjective dimensions of heroin urges: influence of heroin-related and affectively negative stimuli. *Addictive Behaviors*, **14**, 611–623.

Shiffman, S. (1987). Craving: don't let us throw the baby out with the bathwater. *British Journal of Addiction*, **82**, 37–46.

Shiffman, S. & Jarvik, M.E. (1987). Situational determinants of coping in smoking relapse crises. *Journal of Applied Social Psychology*, **17**, 3–15.

Shiffrin, R.M. & Schneider, W. (1977). Controlled and automatic human information processing: II. Perceptual learning, automatic attending, and a general theory. *Psychological Review*, **84**, 127–190.

Southwick, L., Steele, C., Marlatt, A. & Lindell, M. (1981). Alcohol-related expectancies: defined by phase of intoxication and drinking experience. *Journal of Consulting and Clinical Psychology*, **49**, 713–721.

Stewart, J., de Wit, H. & Eikelboom, R. (1984). Role of unconditioned and conditioned drug effects in self-administration of opiates and stimulants. *Psychological Review*, **91**, 251–268.

Tiffany, S.T. (1988). Contempary theories of drug urges, conflicting data, and an alternative cognitive framework. Paper presented at the Conference on Theory and Research in Psychopathology, Performance, and Cognition, Gainsville, FL.

Tiffany, S.T. (1990). A cognitive model of drug urges and drug-use behavior: role of automatic and nonautomatic processes. *Psychological Review*, **97**, 147–168.

Tiffany, S.T. (1991). The application of 1980s psychology to 1990s smoking research. *British Journal of Addiction*, **86**, 617–620.

Tiffany, S.T. (in press). Craving. In *The Macmillan Encyclopedia of Drugs and Alcohol*. New York: Macmillan.

Tiffany, S.T. & Drobes, D.J. (1990). Imagery and smoking urges: the manipulation of affective content. *Addictive Behaviors*, **15**, 531–539.

Tiffany, S.T. & Drobes, D.J. (1991). The development and initial validation of a questionnaire of smoking urges. *British Journal of Addiction*, **86**, 1467–1476.

Tiffany, S.T., Singleton, E., Haertzen, C. & Henningfield, J.E. (1993). The development of a cocaine craving questionnaire. *Drug and Alcohol Dependence*, **34**, 19–28.

Tiffany, S.T., Field, L., Singleton, E., Haertzen, C. & Henningfield, J.E. (1994). The development of a heroin craving questionnaire. Manuscript in preparation.

Tolman, E.C. (1932). *Purposive Behavior in Animals and Men*. New York: Appleton Century.

Tønnesen, P., Nørregaard, J., Simonsen, K. & Sawe, U. (1991). A double-blind trial of a 16-hour transdermal nicotine patch in smoking cessation. *New England Journal of Medicine*, **325**, 311–315.

West, R.J. & Schneider, N. (1987). Craving for cigarettes. *British Journal of Addiction*, **82**, 407–415.

Wetter, D.W., Brandon, T.H. & Baker, T.B. (1992). The relation of affective processing measures and smoking motivation indices among college-age smokers. *Advances in Behaviour Research and Therapy*, **14**, 169–193.

Wills, T.A. & Shiffman, S. (1985). Coping and substance use: a conceptual framework. In S. Shiffman & T.A. Wills (Eds), *Coping and Substance Use*, pp. 3–24. Orlando: Academic Press.

Zinser, M.C., Baker, T.B., Sherman, J.E. & Cannon, D.S. (1992). Relation between self-reported affect and drug urges and cravings in continuing and withdrawing smokers. *Journal of Abnormal Psychology*, **101**, 617–629.

SECTION III

Clinical Applications of Cue Exposure in Addictive Behaviour

CHAPTER 8   Cue exposure treatment in alcohol dependence

Damaris J. Rohsenow[*], *Peter M. Monti*[*] *and David B. Abrams*[**]

Theoretical and empirical work concerning cue reactivity in the addictive disorders, as well as within the obsessive compulsive and phobic disorders, has paved the way to exploring cue exposure techniques to reduce alcoholics' reactions to alcohol cues (Monti et al., 1987; Niaura et al., 1988; Rohsenow et al., 1990). In this chapter we shall briefly review the rationales for cue exposure treatment with alcoholics, consider important methodological issues, examine the pertinent outcome research, and consider directions for future work.

Historically, the rationale for cue exposure treatment has been conceptualized primarily from the perspective of a combination of classical and operant learning models (Hammersley, 1992; Pomerleau, 1981). However, we arrived at cue exposure treatment from a background in social learning theory and cognitive behavior therapy (Monti et al., 1989). This approach was based on the evidence that alcoholics were deficient in alcohol-specific but not general social skills (Abrams et al., 1991; Twentyman et al., 1982), that performance in alcohol-specific role plays but not general role plays predicted treatment success (Monti et al., 1990), that responses to role plays that included alcohol imagery predicted outcome whereas high-risk scenes without drinking cues did not (Goddard et al., 1990), and that alcoholics who were more reactive to alcohol cues had their coping skills more disrupted by the presence of alcohol than did less reactive alcoholics (Binkoff et al., 1984). These results led us to the belief that alcohol cues needed to be incorporated into coping skills training programs with alcoholics. The social learning model has been incorporated into more recent formulations of cue exposure treatment (e.g.

[*]Veterans Affairs Medical Center and Brown University, Providence, Rhode Island, USA
[**]Brown University and the Miriam Hospital, Providence, Rhode Island, USA

Addictive Behaviour: Cue Exposure Theory and Practice.
Edited by D.C. Drummond, S.T. Tiffany, S. Glautier and B. Remington.
© 1995 John Wiley & Sons Ltd.

Marlatt, 1990; Niaura et al., 1988). We will review both the historical and the evolving formulations of the models underlying cue exposure treatment with alcoholics.

As was seen in the earlier chapters, various conditioning models of relapse suggest that environmental and interoceptive cues previously associated with alcohol's effects can elicit a network of conditioned reactions that may play a role in precipitating relapse. Both classical and operant conditioning are thought to be involved in a two-factor model: classical conditioning is used to explain the acquisition of a network of elicited conditioned responses, then an operant conditioning model proposes that the individual emits a response (such as drinking) designed to decrease some aspects of the elicited responses, thus reinforcing the emitted response (Lee & Oei, 1993; Niaura et al., 1988; Pomerleau, 1981).

The conditioning models imply that a series of extinction trials, consisting of non-reinforced exposure to substance use cues, would be helpful in reducing individuals' reactivity. This effect should therefore reduce later craving and relapse when the alcoholic is confronted with alcohol cues. This model has been successfully applied to the treatment of several anxiety disorders. Procedures using cue exposure with response prevention have been explored extensively in the treatment of obsessive compulsive and phobic disorders and have been noted to produce effective outcomes by several reviewers (e.g. Emmelkamp, 1982). A series of studies has empirically investigated parameters of this treatment approach to shed light on factors such as the optimal number of sessions per week, length of sessions, mode of presentation, etc. (e.g. Foa & Kozak, 1986). These treatment methodologies can provide a basis for informed decisions about similar treatment methodologies for alcohol dependence.

Drawing parallels between cue exposure techniques for anxiety-based disorders and for alcohol dependence (Lee & Oei, 1993; Niaura et al., 1988) does not mean that anxiety necessarily underlies alcohol dependence. Rather, any conditioned response is presumed to respond to factors that affect conditioned responses in general. In both types of disorders, conditioned stimuli elicit a set of responses then the client customarily emits a behavior that reduces the conditioned response, resulting in reinforcement of the emitted behavior and a failure to extinguish the elicited response. This framework conceptualizes drinking among alcoholics as similar to compulsive behavior (Hodgson, 1989; Lee & Oei, 1993), and urges to drink and other cognitive reactions to cues as similar to obsessions (Modell et al., 1992). Similar to obsessive compulsive disorders, the alcoholic is troubled by persistent thoughts about drinking in the presence of drinking cues and may feel compelled to drink to reduce the cue-elicited discomfort.

The analogy with anxiety disorders is less exact if during ongoing use alcohol is primarily consumed for its positive reinforcement value, as an appetitive response, rather than for its negative reinforcement value, as an escape response (Baker, Morse & Sherman, 1987; Niaura et al., 1988; Rohsenow et al., 1990; Stewart, de Wit & Eikelboom, 1984). For example, the psychophysiological responses elicited by drinking cues resemble conditioned appetitive motivational responses (Niaura et al., 1988; Rohsenow et al., 1990) unlike the responses to anxiety-eliciting stimuli. However, conditioning principles should still apply to the learned behavior as they apply to any appetitive approach response. The stimuli associated with an appetitive response have been found to produce psychophysiological changes functionally similar to deprivation-induced hunger (Wardle, 1990), so the emitted response may still result in negative reinforcement in addition to positive reinforcement. Treatment is therefore designed to expose the client to the conditioned stimuli to elicit the conditioned response while preventing either the customary emitted response or escape, thereby extinguishing the elicited response.

Extinction of classically conditioned physiological responses is only one mechanism by which cue exposure treatments may reduce drinking. Other mechanisms of action may be involved according to other models, including a broader operant conditioning model and a social learning model of drinking (e.g. Abrams & Niaura, 1987). These mechanisms include a number of cognitive and information processing factors, including breaking the chain of behaviors leading to drinking, disconfirming clients' expectations about the effects of exposure to drinking cues, and strengthening efficacy expectations about their ability to resist drinking in the presence of powerful cues (Abrams & Niaura, 1987; Drummond, Cooper & Glautier, 1990; Niaura et al., 1988; Wilson, 1981). Furthermore, coping skills training conducted in the presence of substance use cues may enhance treatment effectiveness by allowing behavioral rehearsal under environmental and interoceptive conditions more similar to the situational context of high-risk situations in real life. Integrating cue exposure treatments with coping skills training may therefore not only provide more effective practice of skills, but may also be especially effective in promoting outcome expectancies and efficacy expectancies that reduce the probability of drinking. The outcome expectancies involved are the expected effects of experiencing an urge to drink without drinking, which many alcoholics believe would be unbearable. The efficacy expectations involved refer to the person's expected belief that he or she can successfully refrain from drinking when experiencing an urge in the presence of drinking cues.

One controversial methodological issue is centrally tied to these theoretical models. Should limited alcohol ingestion be used as part of the exposure stimuli or would this decrease the effectiveness of the cue exposure sessions? In most treatment facilities, limited alcohol ingestion is not an option due to policy, but it has been used in some studies of cue exposure treatment (e.g. Rankin, Hodgson & Stockwell, 1983) in which harm reduction was the goal. The answer to this question depends on the conceptualization of the conditioned stimulus versus the emitted response which is being prevented. This conceptualization in turn depends on the point in the behavior chain at which the therapist desires the behavior to be interrupted. Theoretically, a set of conditioned stimuli, such as a bad day at work, leads to a network of conditioned responses, primarily affective and psychophysiological (Pomerleau, 1981). In some conceptualizations, drinking is the subsequent emitted response to be prevented. Ingesting any alcohol would provide reinforcement and strengthen the power of the conditioned stimuli to elicit the conditioned response. On the other hand, in some early case studies (Hodgson & Rankin, 1982; Rankin, Hodgson & Stockwell, 1983), controlled drinking was the targeted goal, drinking to intoxication was the response that was being prevented, and the effect of a limited amount of alcohol ingestion was chosen as the targeted conditioned stimulus. Even if drinking more than a certain number of drinks or to intoxication is the emitted response to be prevented, the question remains as to the point in the behavior chain that is more effective in preventing this response. In general, it is easier for a person to interrupt themselves earlier in a behavior chain than closer to the emitted response (Bandura, 1977). Therefore, unless controlled drinking is the client's explicit treatment goal, it is advisable to help clients to interrupt the behavior chain before drinking.

METHODOLOGICAL ISSUES

In this section we shall examine a variety of methodological issues relevant to the design of research studies and to the pertinent elements for effective clinical interventions. The research design issues affect our ability to draw conclusions from the studies available. The clinical issues point to the variety of aspects of the intervention that can vary, and indicate both what is known to date and the size of the task that confronts future researchers.

Research Design Issues

Since cue exposure models for treating alcohol problems are relatively new, there is a paucity of treatment outcome studies on cue exposure treatment with alcoholics. Therefore, issues of study design become crucial when evaluating results.

Single case studies versus group designs

Most of the early publications were case studies that applied cue exposure principles to individual alcoholics and reported the results. When an area is new, single case studies are invaluable in suggesting a direction for controlled research (Kazdin & Wilson, 1978). While the results of single cases provide insights and hypotheses about treatment, the results do not demonstrate a causal relationship between treatment and outcome and are not generalizable across clients (Kazdin & Wilson, 1978). However, although results of single case experimental designs would provide more confidence in the procedure being worthy of further study (Barlow & Hersen, 1984), we know of no study that uses this methodology with cue exposure treatment for alcoholics. The ultimate research design is the randomized controlled experimental between-group design, with a sample size that allows adequate power, and drinking outcome data collected over a follow-up period of adequate length.

Standardization of treatment methodology

In single case studies and some group studies, the therapist is allowed so much flexibility in applying the cue exposure treatment principles that no standardization of treatment procedures is developed. This does not allow separate cases to be compared as the treatment is different, and does not allow others to replicate the methodology and results. After the initial exploratory development stage of a treatment approach it is important for conducting clinical trials to develop standardized treatment manuals that therapists are expected to adhere to, with monitoring of therapist adherence and appropriate feedback.

Follow-up versus post-only designs

Some studies only report the effects of a procedure on target behaviors during the time that treatment is being administered, or only on change from pre- to post-treatment on a standardized measure. This does not provide information about the effects of treatment on the target behavior once the person has completed the treatment, yet this is the most important information.

Process versus outcome measures

The bottom line of an alcohol treatment method is the effect on quantity and/or frequency of drinking and drinking-related problems after treatment completion. However, process measures, either during treatment, as pre–post change measures or during follow-up, can provide information about the effects treatment is having on theoretically relevant mediating mechanisms, such as coping skills or cue reactivity. These measures can be used both in between-group analyses and in correlational analyses of the relationships of process to outcome. Such measures help to improve future treatment methodologies. The benefits of this methodology are illustrated in the treatment outcome studies of Drummond & Glautier (1994) and Monti et al. (1993b) reviewed later in this chapter.

Relevant Cues for Cue Exposure

The nature of the stimuli that a therapist could present can vary widely. One common set of stimuli involves the sight and/or smell of the client's favorite or customary beverage. Conditioning theory indicates that the beverage which is most frequently associated with alcohol's psychophysiological effects is the most relevant conditioned stimulus. A recent parametric laboratory study found that cue reactivity was greater to beverages that were more similar to the individual's usual drink, supporting this hypothesis (Staiger & White, 1991). This study compared desire to drink, withdrawal symptoms and heart rate to the sight and smell of the subject's favorite drink, a similar drink of a different brand, a different type of drink of the same general class (e.g. another hard liquor), a drink of a different class (e.g. presenting beer to a whiskey drinker), and a non-alcoholic drink. Furthermore, the sight and smell of the favorite drink elicited stronger reactions than did the sight alone of the same drink. The issue of whether alcohol consumption should be the stimulus presented was discussed earlier.

Another issue is whether the beverage specific cues are sufficient or whether a broader range of cues, such as affective states, drinking environments, or situations that elicit the motivation to drink, should be presented as well. The sight and smell of the beverage is the final common link in the chain of conditioned stimuli for drinking so intervening at that point may be efficient. However, about 30% of alcoholics we studied failed to react to their customary alcoholic beverage (Rohsenow et al., 1992), a phenomenon also found by other researchers (Cooney et al., 1989). Our experience is that these people can identify situations or events that elicit a strong urge to drink. The behavior chain that leads to drinking commonly has elements that occur before the beverage stimuli appear, including interpersonal and intrapersonal events that elicit mood states that in turn may trigger the motivation to seek out alcohol (see Greeley & Ryan Chapter 6). These elements may be crucial stimuli to target in cue exposure treatment. However, these complex events may be more difficult to present in a controlled manner. A therapist could accompany a client to his living room or to her usual bar, but it is difficult to present the conflict at work or the fight with the client's mother that triggers a drinking episode.

Imaginal versus *in vivo* Exposure to Cues

Directly relevant to the above issue is whether the stimuli can be presented imaginally instead of *in vivo*. For phobics, *in vivo* stimuli are more effective but imaginal presentation of stimuli are equally effective for obsessive compulsives (Foa & Kozak, 1986). Among alcoholics, *in vivo* exposure produced greater changes in response than did imaginal exposure (Rankin, Hodgson & Stockwell, 1983). Since it is easy to present alcoholics with their customary beverage in treatment, *in vivo* exposure at least to the beverage cues should be included. For fairly stable environmental stimuli, either a therapist could accompany the client or the client could be assigned to carry out the exposure *in vivo* as homework (e.g. Blakey & Baker, 1980). A caveat is that the latter may increase the risk of drinking without the presence of someone to help prevent the response.

However, many of the events that trigger drinking bouts, such as marital fights, may be difficult or impossible to present on demand. Furthermore, "it is possible that the critical cues to drug use are primarily in the user's mind rather than in the user's environment" (Hammersley, 1992, p. 299). Imaginal exposure to such high-risk situations, either through visualization or role play, may be the best solution. Clients can also deal with unpredictable situations through homework by giving them a general instruction to practice the exposure with response prevention techniques whenever they experience an urge to drink between sessions.

Another form of imaginal exposure involves mood induction procedures. Mood induction techniques can be used to elevate moods that are commonly associated with drinking or relapse. These techniques have been shown to result in increased urge to drink (Litt el al., 1990; Rubonis et al., 1994). Tying the targeted mood state to the particular situation that commonly induced both the targeted mood and a drinking episode should result in a more effective set of conditioned stimuli. This may be particularly useful with women: while women and men did not differ in their reactivity to beverage cues, women's urge to drink increased more after they received negative affect induction based on their own drinking triggers than did men's (Rubonis et al., 1994).

A recent discussion that integrates the classic tension reduction hypothesis of alcohol abuse (Cappell & Herman, 1972) with classical conditioning goes so far as to propose that the classically conditioned association of negative affect with drug use is less important than negative affect *per se* in motivating drug use (Stasiewicz & Maisto, 1993). This discussion, like Cappell & Herman's (1972), views drug use mainly as an operant response designed to escape or avoid a negative affective state. However, in this view, in addition to providing response extinction to aspects of the stimulus situation that are associated with drinking, extinction of emotional responses *per se* needs to be conducted. This argues that induction of negative moods should be done whether or not the moods have a conditioned association with alcohol use. It may not be possible to extinguish negative moods since affect is part of the human condition, so our own preference is to break the conditioned association between moods and drinking using cue exposure treatment and help clients learn to cope with moods using cognitive behavioral mood management training (Monti et al., 1989, 1995). However, this is an empirical question and the points of Stasiewicz & Maisto (1993) are worth considering.

Individualized versus Standardized Sets of Cues

To what extent should cue exposure approaches be individually tailored to specific clients as opposed to using a standardized set of stimuli? A series of studies with opiate and cocaine abusers has used standardized stimuli (see Dawe & Powell, Chapter 9) but successful work with alcoholics has used either individually tailored sets of stimuli based on initial functional analyses of drinking situations (Blakey & Baker, 1980; Hodgson & Rankin, 1982; Monti et al., 1993b) or a standardized set of cues (Drummond & Glautier, 1994; Rankin, Hodgson & Stockwell, 1983). The individualized approach has been the approach of choice for cue exposure treatment of the anxiety disorders for many years (Foa & Kozak, 1986). Certainly the range of individual differences in cue reactivity (Rees & Heather, Chapter 5) and high-risk situations (Greeley & Ryan, Chapter 6) supports an individualized approach.

Order of Presentation of Cues

Exposure-based treatments have commonly presented conditioned stimuli in a hierarchy. Hodgson (1989) recommended that exposure be graded, presenting the less tempting situations first, then gradually presenting more tempting situations. Drummond & Glautier (1994) used a two-item hierarchy, presenting a less commonly consumed beverage for 5 days then the client's most commonly consumed beverage for the remaining 5 days. As the length of stay in hospitals is uncertain in the current health-care climate in America, we chose to use a modified reverse hierarchy, without difficulty (Monti et al., 1993b). The client's customary beverage stimuli were always presented first each day. Then, while the beverage remained on the table, other drinking-related events were presented imaginally, with the one that provoked the greatest urge to drink being presented first each day (Monti et al., 1993b; Monti et al., 1995). With opiate addicts, the least arousing stimuli were presented first because starting with the mock shoot-up ritual increased dropping out of treatment (A.R. Childress, personal communication, 1988). In treatment of anxiety-based disorders, the ordering of presentation has not been found to be necessary for success, it is simply necessary that exposure occur (e.g. Leitenberg, 1976).

Attention Focus During Cue Exposure Treatment

The aversiveness of cue exposure (Cooney et al., 1987) can lead some clients to cognitively avoid attending to the stimuli or to their elicited responses. This failure to attend could prevent extinction from occurring by minimizing cue reactivity. Two studies instructed subjects with anxiety-based disorders to either focus their attention or distract themselves from cues during cue exposure treatment. Attention-focusing instructions resulted in greater between-sessions habituation (Grayson, Foa & Steketee, 1982; Sartory, Rachman & Grey, 1982). Instructions to focus on their responses may produce even greater cue reactivity than instructions to focus on the stimuli (Lang et al., 1983), which may allow more habituation to occur. Alcoholics who reported attending more to either the stimuli or to their responses during cue exposure assessment drank on fewer days during the next 3 months (Rohsenow et al., 1994). In a social learning formulation, increasing attention to the high-risk situation or responses may allow for greater mobilization of coping resources and decrease the likelihood that automatic overlearned alcohol-seeking responses determine the outcome (Rohsenow et al., 1994; Tiffany, 1990). Thus, attention focus may be therapeutic for several reasons. Laboratory studies of the effects of attention focus on cue reactivity are currently under investigation in our laboratory.

Nature of the Responses Being Monitored

Hierachies of cue situations are most commonly organized on the basis of relative urge or desire to drink or temptation provoked by the situation (e.g. Monti et al., 1993b; Rankin, Hodgson & Stockwell, 1983). Within sessions, the response targeted for monitoring is also usually urge, desire or temptation to drink (e.g. Monti et al., 1993a; Hodgson, 1989). Cue-elicited salivation has been found to be a better predictor of drinking outcome than has urge to drink (Rohsenow et al., 1994). However, salivation would be too difficult to monitor in an ongoing way during treatment sessions. No other psychopysiological response has reliably been elicited by cues except skin conductance (Rohsenow et al., 1990) which would also be difficult to monitor in an ongoing way during cue exposure treatment. Nevertheless, Drummond & Glautier (1994) have successfully monitored skin conductance during a clinical trial and found it to predict latency to initiation of heavy drinking and dependence symptoms. Urge, desire and temptation have the advantage of being easy to monitor and are face-valid, so these constructs are likely to be used until someone can develop a feasible alternative. As long as exposure is occurring, presumably the whole network of conditioned responses is likely to habituate.

Dosage and Regimen

Parametric studies of cue exposure treatment with anxiety-based disorders have found that 50–90 minute sessions of exposure are more effective than shorter sessions, and sessions four or five times per week are more effective than less frequent sessions (e.g. Foa & Kozak, 1986; Marks, 1987). Within-session habituation must occur for treatment to be effective for obsessive compulsives (Foa & Kozak, 1986). It would be reasonable to assume that this will hold true for alcohol cue exposure as well.

Studies of cue exposure treatment with opiate abusers indicate that 1 hour of exposure is more effective than 10 minute sessions of exposure (see Dawe & Powell, Chapter 9). With 10 minute sessions of exposure, craving to cues did not extinguish until after 18 sessions (Childress, McLellan & O'Brien, 1985) while 45 minute sessions resulted in decreased craving after six sessions of cue exposure treatment (Rankin, Hodgson & Stockwell, 1983). In a study in which alcoholics were exposed to the sight and smell of alcohol for 18 minutes followed by continued exposure to the sight of the alcoholic beverage for another 15 minutes, urge to drink peaked at 6 minutes and decreased significantly during the next 12 minutes (Monti et al., 1993a). Urge to drink continued to decrease significantly during the following 15 minutes of visual exposure alone (Rohsenow et al., 1989). Staiger & White (1991) similarly provided 20 consecutive 1 minute trials of the sight and smell of alcohol and found significant decreases in heart rate, desire to drink and withdrawal symptoms. The heart rate change seemed to stabilize within 9 minutes and the self-report measures within 13 minutes. These studies suggest that significant within-session habituation can occur within 18–20 minutes of exposure and can continue to occur while the beverage remains in sight within the room. In controlled treatment trials, six 55 minute trials of exposure resulted in significant decreases in cue reactivity (Monti et al., 1993b), and ten 40 minute trials of exposure in another study produced significant treatment outcome results (Drummond & Glautier, 1994), although the data on pre–post change in cue reactivity have not yet been published for the latter study. Our current recommendations based on the literature of alcohol, cocaine and opiate abusers is that at least six or seven sessions of 45–60 minutes will be needed to be effective.

Timing of Treatment

How long does a client need to be detoxified before cue exposure treatment can start? In the current health-care climate in the US, short lengths of stay may require that cue exposure treatment be initiated before a client is fully detoxified. Recently, no differences were found in magnitude of cue-elicited urge to drink or salivation between alcoholics in their second, fourth or sixth day of unmedicated detoxification, between these groups and alcoholics in their fourth week after their last drink, or between alcoholics receiving detoxification medication and those in unmedicated withdrawal (Monti et al., 1993a). Therefore, the detoxification period seems to result in no abnormal reactivity that would rule out the possibility of conducting cue exposure treatment. However, if clients are taking a medication which is intended to reduce urges to drink or anxiety, it may interfere with extinction by not allowing enough response to be elicited, just as an opioid antagonist has been found to interfere with the effectiveness of cue exposure treatment for anxiety disorders (Merluzzi et al., 1991). Therefore, it may be best to wait until the medication has been discontinued before starting cue exposure treatment if possible.

Setting and Background Treatment

The optimal protection for the client undergoing cue exposure treatment is provided when he or she is an inpatient, as any residual effects of the exposure sessions can be handled therapeutically in a safe environment. However, sufficient length of inpatient stay may not be feasible. After conducting cue exposure assessment or treatment sessions with hundreds of alcohol-dependent clients, not one relapse has been attributed to the exposure procedures, so it may be possible to conduct cue exposure treatment in a less restrictive setting. Furthermore, a benefit of outpatient treatment is the ability of the client to participate in *in vivo* homework assignments (e.g. Blakey & Baker, 1980). However, for cue exposure with response prevention to result in extinction, the emitted response (drinking) must not be occurring between sessions. If the client drinks (or drinks more than the targeted controlled drinking goal), this should prevent extinction from occurring. Therefore, if outpatient treatment is to be conducted, the client should make a commitment to the treatment goal, the therapist should assess the abstinence or adherence to the goal in some way at the start of every session, and the cue exposure treatment should terminate if the client has failed to adhere to the abstinence or the controlled drinking goal.

A somewhat related issue is that cue exposure treatment is not intended to be the sole form of treatment for alcohol abuse. Alcohol abuse and dependence is a complex problem and needs to be addressed within the context of a complete treatment program. If other contributing issues are not dealt with, such as vocational, psychiatric, medical, family, and social needs, these may precipitate relapse. However, cue exposure treatment may provide a useful adjunct to a comprehensive alcohol treatment program by addressing an important aspect of recovery that is not commonly treated.

Passive Exposure versus Active Coping Approaches

In the classical conditioning model, a series of cue exposure trials should result in extinction of the conditioned response. Urge to drink was seen to decrease over one extended trial of simple exposure (Monti et al., 1993a) and over a series of repeated trials of exposure (Drummond & Glautier, 1994; Rankin, Hodgson & Stockwell, 1983; Staiger & White, 1991). However, clinical trials of cue exposure treatment with opiate abusers suggest that generalization may not occur from cues used in the sessions to other cues in the environment (Childress et al., 1988). A social learning approach would suggest that a more comprehensive approach to cue exposure would be preferable (Marlatt, 1990; Monti et al., 1989). It is possible that teaching active coping strategies during cue exposure may be more effective for several reasons. First, passive exposure to drinking cues is quite aversive and could lead to greater attrition if clients did not expect to learn more active tools during the sessions. Learning coping strategies during cue exposure makes clinical sense to our clients. Second, alcoholics who are more reactive to drinking cues also have their coping skills more disrupted in the presence of alcohol (Binkoff et al., 1984). Skills training in the presence of the cues may decrease the disruptive effects of the cues on the execution of coping skills. It may be that a form of state-dependent learning occurs such that an alcoholic needs to practice coping skills while in the altered psychophysiological state produced by the drinking cues. Third, any strong motivation such as urge to drink may result in a narrowing of attention (Sayette et al., 1995) and impaired coping skills (Hodgson, 1989). If this is so, then coping skills may need to be practiced under similar motivational conditions so the client can learn to cope with the situation while experiencing such "tunnel vision" (Hodgson, 1989). Fourth, coping skills training was incorporated into several of the early pilot studies of cue exposure treatment (Blakey & Baker, 1980; Hodgson, 1989; Rankin, Hodgson & Stockwell, 1983) and may partially account for some of the positive results. For these reasons, urge coping skills training has been incorporated into cue exposure treatment approaches by several groups of researchers (Childress, 1993; Cooney et al., 1993; Monti et al., 1993b). However, it is important that exposure continues throughout the coping skills training for optimal effectiveness within this model.

TREATMENT STUDIES

Single Case Studies

Pickens, Bigelow & Griffiths (1973) report perhaps the earliest published case of cue exposure with an alcoholic client. Cue exposure was used in the third of four treatment phases designed to alter the maladaptive disciminative control that had been acquired over drinking for a 29 year old unmarried male alcoholic. Following an initial 6 week phase of free access to alcohol and a second experimental phase during which contingencies between alcoholic drinking and socialization were successfully revised, a third experimental phase began in which the researchers altered some of the stimulus control of drinking by using a stimulus fading procedure. This entailed presenting the client with stimuli that were more and more closely associated with drinking until he no longer wanted a drink. Stimulus presentation was arranged immediately before some scheduled activity such as meal times, thus decreasing the probability that it would trigger a drinking episode. Eventually drinking itself was presented. The client was initially required to simply sniff bourbon and later to taste and drink it. In the latter part of the fading procedure, when full 1 ounce drinks were used, the client was told to decrease the magnitude of each sip and increase the time between sips. Sip magnitude gradually decreased over time as did the rate of drinking. In a fourth treatment phase, an attempt was made to establish alternative reinforcers to maintain non-drinking behavior, and several months later the client was placed on Antabuse. The authors reported that at a 1 year follow-up the client was employed full-time with no drinking-related absences from work. However, no drinking data are reported at follow-up and given the multifaceted treatment approach, it is difficult to assess the effect of cue exposure in this study. Nevertheless, the authors are to be credited for their innovative achievements.

Hodgson & Rankin (1976) report the case of a 43 year old male with a 26 year history of abusive drinking who presented for treatment at the Maudsley Hospital, the site for much of the pioneering work in cue exposure treatment. Although the authors report that several drinking cues were identified, since alcohol itself was the strongest, they decided to use a priming dose of either one double vodka (40 ml 65.5% proof) or four double vodkas (apparently depending upon the treatment day). The procedure involved initial testing at approximately 10.30 h followed by the priming dose, which the client was encouraged to drink as quickly as possible. After consuming the drink the client returned to his room where he relaxed and participated in hourly assessments. During this time alcohol was always available. Thus, response prevention was "very gentle and involved no physical coercion" (p. 215).

The initial results of treatment showed that the client's desire for a drink extinguished across treatment days. In addition, the authors report that while the client expected that the response prevention period would be very distressing, this expectation was modified by the treatment. The final stage of the 4 week treatment period involved consumption of eight vodkas (320 ml) in 1 hour in order to induce feelings of intoxication that would normally have resulted in further drinking. While craving did increase slightly, it apparently returned to baseline within 4 hours.

The most unique aspect of this case study is the fact that the follow-up period lasted for 6 years. During the first 6 months of this period the client reported six drinking occasions, none lasting more than 1 day. Both the client and his wife confirmed that the six occasions were atypical in that drinking and stopping had never occurred during the 3 year period preceding treatment. The authors construed the client's unscheduled drinking sessions as *in vivo* cue exposure practice and reinforced this view by telling the client, as reported in a later chapter (Hodgson & Rankin, 1982), "Although you feel that you failed, we would like you to look at your lapses in rather a different way. What you are proving to yourself is that when you do start drinking, you are no longer totally helpless. You are now able to stop even after a heavy drinking session, so that 'one drink, one drunk' no longer applies to you" (p. 217). The authors report that over the next $5\frac{1}{2}$ years the number of heavy drinking days (a day on which more than 100 g of alcohol was consumed) was drastically reduced from pretreatment. Hodgson & Rankin concluded that the client"s changed self-control strategies and perceived self-efficacy positively influenced his pattern of consumption.

In another single case study originating from the Maudsley Hospital, Rankin (1982) reports on a chronic male alcoholic treated with cue exposure and response prevention. Following an experimental phase designed to test drinking rate (which had been shown to correlate with craving or disposition to drink) the client received six treatment sessions on alternate days (excluding weekends). Treatment was followed by a second test phase. Treatment included the client sitting at a table on which there was a bottle of his preferred alcoholic beverage and a glass. Next, for three 15 minute phases, the client was asked—for consecutive 3 minutes periods—to hold the beverage glass, maintain eye contact with it, and hold it to his mouth so that he could smell the alcohol. The client was instructed, "The idea of treatment is to resist the drink. However, if you find it impossible to resist, then you can drink it—the idea is to resist it if you can" (p. 236). Following discharge from the hospital the client was given cue exposure with response prevention tasks including watching television with a bottle in front of him with the instruction that he could have no more than one double scotch and going into a pub and just ordering one double when he was feeling tense.

Results of the inpatient phases showed reduction on self-reported measures of "desire", "difficulty to resist", and "temptation", for both test phases and treatment sessions. In addition, latency to consume the test doses in the pre- and post-treatment tests showed differences from 592 to 999 seconds. Results of the outpatient treatment were similarly successful in that there was a decrease in the difficulty rating of the assignments. At a 9 month follow-up the client was reported to be drinking not more than two pints of beer at a time, and only at lunchtime or on Sundays in the pub. Furthermore, he reported no desire to increase consumption and much improved family relationships. The author suggests that treatment effected change through a change in cognitions that was brought about by the disconfirmation of negative expectancies purported to occur after successful resistance to alcohol. The major contribution of this clinical report is its utilization of *in vivo* self-paced homework and its theoretical discussion related to self-efficacy. While the controlled drinking goal adapted in this case may be controversial for some readers, it should be emphasized that abstinence is also an entirely appropriate goal for cue exposure work.

In what seems to be the first report of combining cue exposure treatment with coping skills training, Blakey & Baker (1980) studied six chronic but motivated alcoholic male clients ranging from 36 to 49 years of age. This series of case studies also differs from those previously reported in that the treatment goal was abstinence and thus exposure did not involve consuming alcohol: an important conceptual, methodological and clinical point, as emphasized earlier. The treatment was individualized for each client and involved exposing each client to his favorite drink in a variety of settings including both laboratory and naturalistic drinking environments. The amount of exposure seemed to vary considerably and not all clients received coping skills training. Coping skills training, when conducted, generally involved clients role playing dealing with difficult situations, including drink refusal skills, listing alternative activities and reinforcing self-control. Nevertheless, the treatment proved effective in four out of the six clients in that these four were abstinent at between 2 and 9 months follow-up. The authors concluded that the treatment was successful and that it warranted further study.

Group Design Studies

The first randomized group clinical trial of cue exposure treatment was conducted by Rankin, Hodgson & Stockwell (1983). Ten severely alcohol-dependent male clients were randomly assigned to either six cue exposure plus response prevention sessions using *in vivo* exposure to alcohol, or to a comparison treatment consisting of six imaginal exposure sessions, followed by six *in vivo* cue exposure plus response prevention sessions. All clients were hospitalized and had been abstinent 7–10 days prior to treatment. In a pre-treatment session all clients received a prim-ing dose of alcohol in which they drank two drinks over the course of 20 minutes. Upon finishing drinking and 15, 30 and 45 minutes after, subjective measures such as desire to drink and difficulty resisting drink-ing as well as measures of breath alcohol level, pulse, and tremor were recorded. After recording the last measure of the 45 minutes interval, two drinks of the client's preferred alcoholic beverage were poured and the client was instructed to drink them *ad lib*. Assessment measures were repeated following treatment. In the *in vivo* exposure trials, a third drink was poured with the instruction that the client was to resist further drinking. These trials involved clients holding and smelling a glass of their favorite drink for 3 minutes at 15 minutes intervals and maintaining eye contact with it otherwise. Experimental sessions were approximately 45 minutes in duration. They consisted of following the priming dose of alcohol with the instruction, "I am now going to pour a third drink. The idea of treatment is that you resist this drink. However, if you find it impossible to resist then you can drink it—the idea is to resist if you can" (p. 437). In the comparison condition clients were asked to imagine being exposed to alcohol during the same period and to imagine success-fully refusing the drink and using coping skills. As the comparison con-dition used imaginal cue exposure with coping skills rehearsal, it was designed to compare two methods of conducting cue exposure treatment rather than to control for non-specific treatment factors *per se*.

Results of this study showed that *in vivo* cue exposure ($n = 10$) resulted in a decrease in desire for alcohol and difficulty in resisting a drink across treatment sessions while the imaginal exposure sessions ($n = 5$) resulted in trivial decreases. Furthermore, after *in vivo* exposure clients drank more slowly in the timed drinking test while clients receiving imaginal exposure did not, and this was interpreted as an indication of less crav-ing. Interestingly, the measures of pulse and tremor, while increased dur-ing cue exposure, did not show a decrement across sessions and did not differentiate the types of exposure. Unfortunately, this study reported no follow-up data. Furthermore, this study had a very small sample size which means it may have had insufficient power to detect effects of the imaginal exposure, and it limits the generalizability of the results.

In a preliminary study recently published from our laboratory (Monti et al., 1993b), we have investigated the combined effectiveness of cue exposure with urge coping skills training. Thirty-four alcoholic male cli-ents hospitalized at a Veterans Affairs Medical Center and receiving standard alcohol treatment were randomly assigned to receive either the experimental treatment or no additional treatment. All clients had been diagnosed alcohol dependent according to DSM-III-R criteria (American

Psychiatric Association, 1987), had a goal of abstinence, and received the standard inpatient alcoholism treatment program.

The experimental treatment consisted of six individually administered 1 hour treatment sessions that had three basic goals: (1) to teach the client to identify high-risk situations that result in increased urge to drink; (2) to expose the client to these triggers during treatment until urge to drink had decreased; and (3) to teach specific coping strategies to deal with urge to drink in high-risk situations. The rationale presented to the client was that since many alcoholics react to triggers associated with drinking with a greater urge to drink, and since triggers cannot always be avoided, the treatment was designed to teach clients to handle reactions to triggers. Clients were told that the program was designed to help them build their coping skills so that they could resist temptation more easily and that this would be accomplished by asking them to experience their triggers until they felt their urge to drink decreasing. The contrast group received no additional treatment, only daily evaluations of urge to drink.

Treatment sessions were administered on consecutive days excluding weekends and always began with exposure to the client's customary beverage(s), prepared in the way that he usually consumed it. The client was asked to pour and mix the drink, then to handle and/or sniff it (unless sniffing caused urge to decrease), while reporting his changes in urge to drink. Intensive beverage focus was continued until the client's urge was minimal. Approximately 5–15 minutes at the beginning of each session were spent focusing intensively on the beverage. However, the beverage remained before them throughout the 55 minute sessions, and clients often handled the beverage while imagining trigger situations. Next clients were asked to imagine experiencing their most difficult and/or frequent drinking trigger. Clients were asked to report their urge to drink every time it changed. When the urge had reached its highest point (according to both therapist and client), clients were asked to practice one of several coping strategies while imagining still being in the high-risk situation. The scene was terminated when urge was minimal.

Coping methods were first described, then practiced by having clients imagine using the method while in a high-risk situation. The urge coping strategies that were taught included:

- passive delay and delay as a cognitive strategy
- negative consequences of drinking
- positive consequences of sobriety
- urge reduction imagery
- consummatory substitution

- behavioral substitution
- cognitive mastery statements
- pleasant imagery environments.

See Monti et al. (1995) for details of each of these coping strategies. Clients were given homework assignments to anticipate and practice coping with urges between sessions.

Clients in both conditions participated in pre- and post-treatment assessments that included paper and pencil measures as well as our cue reactivity assessment (Monti et al., 1987, 1993a). Among clients who had reacted to alcohol cues pre-treatment, those who received cue exposure treatment decreased more in urge to drink than did the standard care group.

Those clients who had received the experimental treatment had a higher incidence of abstinence and a higher percentage of abstinent days during the 3–6 months post-treatment than those who had received the standard treatment alone. Groups did not differ in latency to first drink or to heavy drinking. Furthermore, 3 and 6 month follow-up interviews showed that clients who received cue exposure treatment used the coping strategies of thinking about the negative consequences of drinking and the positive consequences of sobriety more than clients in the standard care group. Use of the strategies was significantly related to improvement in quantity and frequency of drinking. These findings are consistent with the notion that cue exposure clients learned coping skills that they applied over time while the positive effects of standard care alone diminished. Upon closer examination it was found that some of the cue exposure clients who drank during the first 3 months post-treatment were completely abstinent during the next 3 months. This was interpreted as supporting the notion that these clients applied coping skills after lapsing and as not supporting an extinction-based hypothesis.

Based on the promising results of our preliminary investigations, we are currently undertaking a much larger scale controlled trial of cue exposure treatment and coping skills training (Monti, 1993). Cue exposure treatment was administered as described for the previous study and as reported in Monti et al. (1993b). While this clinical trial is still ongoing, preliminary results with half the sample completed lend additional support to the notion of combining cue exposure with coping skills training. In this clinical trial, both male and female alcoholic clients, diagnosed according to DSM-III-R criteria for alcohol dependence, who were residing in a residential private facility for alcoholism treatment, were randomly assigned to one of four experimental conditions:

1. Cue exposure plus coping skills training;
2. Cue exposure plus general alcohol education;
3. Relaxation training plus coping skills training; or
4. Relaxation training plus general alcohol education.

All clients participated in extensive assessment batteries at both pre- and post-treatment including cue reactivity assessment. See Monti et al. (1993a) for details of the cue reactivity assessment protocol. Results at our 3 month post-discharge follow-up showed that fewer clients who had received cue exposure plus coping skills training had relapsed to alcohol and fewer had returned to heavy drinking than had those in the other treatment groups.

In another recently reported controlled trial of cue exposure treatment, Drummond & Glautier (1994) studied 35 hospitalized male clients who were referred to an alcoholic clinic for treatment. All clients were diagnosed alcohol dependent according to DSM-III-R criteria (American Psychiatric Association, 1987) and all had a goal of abstinence. Clients were sequentially assigned to either a cue exposure condition or to a relaxation control condition in addition to standard inpatient treatment. Cue exposure clients were told the purpose of the study was to assess whether exposure to the sight and smell of alcohol would be a helpful treatment and that treatment could be used to help them gain confidence in resisting drinking. Clients were asked not to drink the alcohol which was presented to them for 40 minute sessions on 10 weekdays. Clients were instructed to "act out drinking" by picking the drink up, looking at it, smelling it and thinking about it.

Control clients also received some cue exposure, but only one-twentieth of the exposure group's dose. Control clients were given the same rationale for the cue exposure element of their treatment, but were also told that difficulty with tension was a common reason for relapse. Thus, they also received relaxation training. All clients participated in a cue reactivity test on days 1, 5, 6 and 10. This involved both self-report and psychophysiological assessment response to both low and high salience favorite alcoholic beverages.

The results of this study, that included a 6 month follow-up interval, showed that the cue exposure clients did better than the controls in terms of latency to reinstatement of heavy drinking and dependence and in quantity consumed. There were no between-group differences in terms of latency to first drink, or in the number of clients abstinent over the follow-up period. Interestingly, regression analyses showed that treatment group and cue reactivity independently predicted outcome in terms of latency to reinstatement of heavier drinking and dependence. Thus, the authors suggest that the mechanisms of cue exposure may be more complex that than proposed by a learning model that relies exclusively on reactivity. They go on to speculate that perhaps their clients developed increased self-efficacy and were able to use effective coping skills in resisting heavier drinking once drinking began, a conclusion similar to that reached by Monti et al. (1993b) in the previously reported study. Furthermore, Drummond & Glautier suggest that their treatment effects might be enhanced by encouraging the learning of specific cognitive coping in the presence of alcohol cues. While this study has many strengths, perhaps its greatest contribution lies in its analysis of outcome in terms of latency to drinking at increasing levels, particularly as this view has both practical and theoretical implications.

Several other controlled clinical trials are currently underway. Staiger et al. (1993) provided 50 alcohol-dependent males with ten 20 minute trials of exposure to either alcohol (experimental group) or juice (control group). In the post-treatment cue reactivity assessment, the cue exposure group swallowed less (a measure of salivation) than the control group. Preliminary analyses indicate more people abstinent in the experimental group (66%) than in the control group (44%) at 12 months follow-up.

Consistent with the recommendations of several researchers in the field (e.g. Monti et al., 1989; Drummond & Glautier, 1994), Pead et al. (1993) are in the process of conducting a controlled trial of cognitive behavioral skills training alone versus in combination with *in vivo* cue exposure treatment. This trial extends previous work particularly in its attempt to amplify the generalizability of cue situations. Pead et al. suggest that sustained group-based exposure provides a more realistic approximation of real life alcohol exposure than brief individual exposures. Indeed, this study involves 9 weeks of aftercare that include outings with therapists to potential high-risk environments such as bars and restaurants. The results of this trial should provide the field with a good test of the efficacy of real life cue exposure and coping skills training.

Cooney et al. (1993) also are in the process of conducting a large-scale controlled clinical trial of cue exposure combined with urge coping skills training, similar to that described by Monti et al. (1995). In this two-group design, all clients are receiving coping skills training and half are receiving six sessions of cue exposure treatment, all administered in individual sessions. Changes in cue reactivity are being assessed before and after treatment, and follow-up interviews are done 3 and 6 months after treatment. As 86 clients will enter the study, the results should be informative.

Thus, the current research trend involves controlled clinical trials with a range of drinking data collected at follow-up. Furthermore, cue exposure treatment is increasingly being conducted in combination with coping skills training. The results of current ongoing trials should provide valuable information about this combined treatment approach.

FUTURE DIRECTIONS

Research on cue exposure treatment for alcohol-dependent people is in its infancy. The results of the few case studies and controlled studies have been promising, but most of the research in this area has yet to be done. For these reasons, it would be premature for us to recommend that cue exposure be put routinely into practice in treatment programs.

Most of the clinical issues brought up in the methodologies section have yet to be evaluated within the context of cue exposure treatment with alcoholics although some have been investigated in analog studies. Controlled experimental studies are needed of the relative effectiveness of various types of cues to use in treatment, of imaginal versus *in vivo* presentiation of stimuli, of individually tailored versus standardized stimuli, of limited alcohol ingestion as part of the stimulus exposure, of the use of various hierarchies, of different types of attention focus, of monitoring urge as opposed to other responses, of length and number of sessions, of timing and setting of treatment, and of passive exposure alone versus exposure combined with coping skills training.

Ways to match clients to cue exposure treatment need to be investigated further. Across our studies, about 30% of our alcoholic clients fail to react to alcohol cues with increased urge to drink, and a similar percentage fail to react with increased salivation (Rohsenow et al., 1992). Only those clients who demonstrate cue reactivity would be expected to be affected by cue exposure treatment, a hypothesis that was supported by data of Monti et al. (1993b). Many other client variables could be investigated that may interact with cue exposure treatment, such as attentional factors (Rohsenow et al., 1994; Sayette et al., 1995), reactivity to mood induction (Rubonis et al., 1994), family history of alcohol problems (Drummond & Glautier, 1994), gender (Rubonis et al., 1994), co-morbidity of mood disorders (Rubonis et al., 1994), and use of other substances (Gulliver et al., 1995).

Another issue is how to deal with a lapse during the course of cue exposure treatment. If conditioning principles underlie the effects of cue exposure, then response prevention should be absolute for extinction to occur. If the response that should be prevented (either drinking or drinking beyond a certain limit) occurs, should the cue exposure program start over from the beginning? Or would it be better to switch to a different form of treatment and discontinue cue exposure at that point? These issues must be thoughtfully planned before initiating cue exposure treatment with outpatients.

It is clear that cue exposure treatment can be applied within either an abstinence or a controlled drinking (harm reduction) framework. However, it is important to note that the controlled group design studies have all been conducted within an abstinence framework. Thus it is still an empirical question as to whether cue exposure treatment will ultimately be effective within a harm reduction framework. As there is no evidence from controlled clinical trials to support the administration of alcohol during cue exposure treatment, we cannot recommend it at this time.

Given the recent interest in the promising results of clinical trials of various pharmacological adjuncts such as opiate antagonists with alcoholics (e.g. O'Malley et al., 1992), additional directions include issues such as the effects of various medications on the effectiveness of cue exposure when cue exposure treatment and medications are given either sequentially or simultaneously. Would an opiate antagonist interfere with the ability to elicit an alcohol cue reactivity response and thus prevent cue exposure treatment from being effective, just as it interferes with cue exposure treatment for anxiety disorders (Merluzzi et al., 1991)? It may be preferable to conduct cue exposure treatment without medication first, then use an opiate antagonist during the following outpatient weeks to give the clients additional support during the time that they are at highest risk for relapse. Such a clinical trial is currently being planned in our laboratory. Issues concerning the use of disulfiram also need to be carefully considered. Could a client have a disulfiram reaction from sniffing the alcohol? Should alternative cues such as pictures or only imaginal exposure therefore be used, or would these not have sufficient stimulus value? Could disulfiram create a different expectancy set so that clients would not be tempted by alcohol cues while on disulfiram, only to be vulnerable after disulfiram has been discontinued? Other medications may interfere with the ability to elicit a response. A client on haloperidol will fail to show a response to a priming dose of alcohol (Modell et al., 1993) but there is no evidence about the effects of most other medications on elicited responses.

The types of treatment outcome measures collected can allow predictions more closely tailored to theory, as Drummond & Glautier (1994) showed. By investigating latency to return to various levels of drinking, the extent to which the treatment results corresponded to different learning theory predictions could be investigated. The extinction model predicts that cue exposure treatment would decrease the probability of any drinking (Niaura et al., 1988) and increase latency to first drink (Drummond & Glautier, 1994). However, cue exposure treatment should have no effect on any variable related to amount of drinking after the initial lapse reinstates the extinguished response (Drummond & Glautier, 1994). By collecting data on latency to heavier drinking as well as to initial drinking, they were able to suggest that extinction was unlikely to have mediated the beneficial treatment outcomes found. Furthermore, collecting and reporting drinking outcome data for consecutive blocks of time during follow-up also sheds light on mechanisms. Cue exposure treatment resulted in differences in abstinent days during the second 3 months, not the first 3 months after treatment, which is consistent with a coping skills explanation but not with an extinction model of treatment effects (Monti et al., 1993b). Thus, a diversity of outcome measures will allow us to advance both theory and clinical practice.

As can be seen, work on cue exposure treatment is still in its infancy. At this point, no one definitive treatment approach and no one definitive study can be recommended. However, the initial exploratory stage has been completed, and the legion of controlled experimental studies that are needed are just beginning. A few years ago, Heather & Bradley (1990) asked "why are we waiting" for controlled clinical trials of cue exposure treatment. Now, their challenge is being answered.

REFERENCES

Abrams, D.B. & Niaura, R.S. (1987). Social learning theory. In H.T. Blane & K.E. Leonard (Eds), *Psychological Theories of Drinking and Alcoholism*. pp. 131–178. New York: Guilford.

Abrams, D.B., Binkoff, J.A., Zwick, W.R., Liepman, M.R., Nirenberg, T.D., Munroe, S.M. & Monti, P.M. (1991). Alcohol abusers' and social drinkers' responses to alcohol-relevant and general situations. *Journal of Studies on Alcohol*, **52**, 409–414.

American Psychiatric Association (1987). *Diagnostic and Statistical Manual*, 3rd edn, revised. Washington, DC: American Psychiatric Association.

Baker, T.B., Morse, E. & Sherman, J.E. (1987). The motivation to use drugs: a psychobiological analysis of urges. In C. Rivers (Ed.), *The Nebraska Symposium on Motivation: Alcohol Use and Abuse*, pp. 257–323. Lincoln, NE: University of Nebraska Press.

Bandura, A. (1977). *Social Learning Theory*. Englewood Cliffs, NJ: Prentice Hall.

Barlow, D.H. & Hersen, M. (1984). *Single Case Experimental Designs: Strategies for Studying Behavior Change*, 2nd edn. New York: Pergamon Press.

Binkoff, J.A., Abrams, D.B., Collins, R.L., Liepman, M.R., Monti, P.M., Nirenberg, T.D. & Zwick, W.R. (1984). Exposure to alcohol cues: impact of reactivity and drink refusal skills in problem and non-problem drinkers. Paper presented at the Annual Conference of the Association for the Advancement of Behavior Therapy, Philadelphia, PA.

Blakey, R. & Baker, R. (1980). An exposure approach to alcohol abuse. *Behaviour Research and Therapy*, **18**, 319–325.

Cappell, H. & Herman, C.P. (1972). Alcohol and tension reduction: A review. *Quarterly Journal of Studies on Alcohol*, **33**, 33–64.

Childress, A.R. (1993). Using active strategies to cope with cocaine cue reactivity: preliminary treatment outcomes. Paper presented at the NIDA Technical Review Meeting, "Treatment of Cocaine Dependence: Outcome Research". Bethesda, MD, September.

Childress, A.R., McLellan, A.T. & O'Brien, C.P. (1985). Assessment and extinction of conditioned withdrawal-like responses in an integrated treatment for opiate dependence. In L.S. Harris (Ed.), *Problems of Drug Dependence, 1984*, National Institute of Drug Abuse Research Monograph 55, pp. 202–210. Washington, DC: US Government Printing Office.

Childress, A.R., McLellan, A.T., Ehrman, R. & O'Brien, C.P. (1988). Conditioned craving and arousal in cocaine addiction: a preliminary report. Presented at the National Institute on Drug Abuse CPDD Meeting, Philadelphia, PA, June.

Colby, S.M., Gulliver, S.B., Rohsenow, D.J., Monti, P.M., Niaura, R.S., Abrams, D.B., Sirota, A.D., Rubonis, A.V. & Michalec, E. (1991). Impact of alcohol cue reactivity on the smoking topography of male alcoholics. Poster presented at the Annual Meeting of the Association for Advancement of Behavior Therapy, New York, November.

Cooney, N.L., Gillespie, R.A., Baker, L.H. & Kaplan, R.F. (1987). Cognitive changes after alcohol cue exposure. *Journal of Consulting and Clinical Psychology*, **55**, 150–155.

Cooney, N.L., Litt, M.D., Agupp, L. & Schmidt, P.M. (1989). Recent attempts to increase alcohol cue reactivity in alcoholics: the effect of negative moods. In D.J. Rohsenow (Chair), "Recent advances in cue reactivity research in the addictions". Symposium presented at the Annual Meeting of the Association for Advancement of Behavior Therapy, Washington, DC, November.

Cooney, N.L., Bastone, E.C., Schmidt, P.M., Litt, M.D., Bauer, L.O. & Kadden, R. (1993). Cue exposure treatment for alcohol dependence: process and outcome results. In P.M. Monti (Chair), "Cue exposure and alcohol treatment: where do we stand?" Symposium conducted at the Sixth International Conference on Treatment of Addictive Behaviors, Santa Fe, NM.

Drummond, D.C. & Glautier, S.P. (1994). A controlled trial of cue exposure treatment in alcohol dependence. *Journal of Consulting and Clinical Psychology*, **62**, 809–817.

Drummond, D.C., Cooper, T. & Glautier, S.P. (1990). Conditioned learning in alcohol dependence: implications for cue exposure treatment. *British Journal of Addiction*, **85**, 725–743.

Emmelkamp, P. (1982) *Phobic and Obsessive-Compulsive Disorder*. New York: Plenum.

Foa, E.B. & Kozak, M.J. (1986). Emotional processing of fear: exposure to corrective information. *Psychological Bulletin*, **99**, 20–35.

Goddard, P., Rubonis, A.V., Rohsenow, D.J., Monti, P.M. & Abrams, D.B. (1990). Problem-solving skills in alcoholics: a preliminary investigation. Presented at the Annual Meeting of the Midwestern Psychological Association, Chicago, May.

Grayson, J.G., Foa, E.B. & Steketee, G. (1982). Habituation during exposure treatment: distraction vs. attention-focusing. *Behaviour Research and Therapy*, **20**, 323–328.

Gulliver, S.B., Rohsenow, D.J., Colby, S.M., Dey, A.N., Abrams, D.B., Niaura, R.S. & Monti, P.M. (1995). Interrelationship of smoking and alcohol dependence, use and urges to use. *Journal of Studies on Alcohol*, in press.

Hammersley, R. (1992). Cue exposure and learning theory. *Addictive Behaviors*, **17**, 297–300.

Heather, N. & Bradley, B.P. (1990). Cue exposure as a practical treatment for addictive disorders: why are we waiting? *Addictive Behaviors*, **15**, 335–337.

Hodgson, R.J. (1989). Resisting temptation: a psychological analysis. *British Journal of Addiction*, **84**, 251–257.

Hodgson, R.J. & Rankin, H.J. (1976). Modification of excessive drinking by cue exposure. *Behaviour Research and Therapy*, **14**, 305–307.

Hodgson, R.J. & Rankin, H.J. (1982). Cue exposure and relapse prevention. In P. Nathan and W. Hay (Eds), *Case Studies in the Behavioral Modification of Alcoholism*, pp. 207–226. New York. Plenum Press.

Kazdin, A.E. & Wilson, G.T. (1978). *Evaluation of Behavior Therapy: Issues, Evidence, and Research Strategies*, p. 166. New York: Ballinger.

Lang, P.J., Levin, D.N., Miller, G.A. & Kozak, M.J. (1983). Fear behavior, fear imagery, and the psychophysiology of emotion: the problem of affective response integration. *Journal of Abnormal Psychology*, **92**, 276–306.

Lee, N.K. & Oei, T.P.S. (1993). Exposure and response prevention in anxiety disorders: Implications for treatment and relapse prevention in problem drinkers. *Clinical Psychology Review*, **13**, 619–632.

Leitenberg, H. (1976). Behavioral approaches to treatment of neuroses. In H. Leitenberg (Ed.), *Handbook of Behavior Modification and Behavior Therapy*. New York: Prentice Hall.

Litt, M.D., Cooney, N.L., Kadden, R.M. & Gaupp, L. (1990). Reactivity to alcohol cues and induced moods in alcoholics. *Addictive Behaviors*, **15**, 137–146.

Marks, I.M. (1987). *Fears, Phobias and Rituals: Panic, Anxiety and their Disorders*. New York: Oxford University Press.

Marlatt, G.A. (1990). Cue exposure and relapse prevention in the treatment of addictive behaviors. *Addictive Behaviors*, **15**, 395–399.

Merluzzi, T.V., Taylor, C.B., Boltwood, M. & Gotestam, K.G. (1991). Opioid antagonist impedes exposure. *Journal of Consulting and Clinical Psychology*, **59**, 425–430.

Modell, J.G., Glaser, F.B., Mountz, J.M., Schmaltz, S. & Cyr, L. (1992). Obsessive and compulsive characteristics of alcohol abuse and dependence: quantification by a newly developed questionnaire. *Alcoholism: Clinical and Experimental Research*, **16**, 266–271.

Modell, J.G., Mountz, J.M., Glaser, F.B. & Lee, J.Y. (1993). Effect of haloperidol on measures of craving and impaired control in alcoholic subjects. *Alcoholism: Clinical and Experimental Research*, **17**, 234–240.

Monti, P.M. (1993). Craving for relapse. Paper presented to the American Society of Addiction Medicine Annual Meeting, Los Angeles, CA.

Monti, P.M., Binkoff, J.A., Abrams, D.B., Zwick, W.R., Nirenberg, T.D. & Liepman, M.R. (1987). Reactivity of alcoholics and nonalcoholics to drinking cues. *Journal of Abnormal Psychology*, **96**, 122–126.

Monti, P.M., Abrams, D.B., Kadden, R.M. & Cooney, N.L. (1989). *Treating Alcohol Dependence: A Coping Skills Training Guide*, New York: Guilford Press.

Monti, P.M., Abrams, D.B., Binkoff, J.A., Zwick, W.R., Liepman, M.R., Nirenberg,

T.D. & Rohsenow, D.J. (1990). Communication skills training with family, and cognitive-behavioral mood management training for alcoholics. *Journal of Studies on Alcohol*, **51**, 263–270.

Monti, P.M., Rohsenow, D.J., Rubonis, A.V., Niaura, R.S., Sirota, A.D., Colby, S.M. & Abrams, D.B. (1993a). Alcohol cue reactivity: effects of detoxification and extended exposure. *Journal of Studies on Alcohol*. **54**, 235–245.

Monti, P.M., Rohsenow, D.J., Rubonis, A.V., Niaura, R.S., Sirota, A.D., Colby, S.M., Goddard, P. & Abrams, D.B. (1993b). Cue exposure with coping skills treatment for male alcoholics: a preliminary investigation. *Journal of Consulting and Clinical Psychology*, **61**, 1011–1019.

Monti, P.M., Rohsenow, D.J., Colby, S.M. & Abrams, D.B. (1995). Coping and social skills training. In R.K. Hester and W.R. Miller (Eds), *Handbook of Alcoholism Treatment Approaches*, 2nd edn. New York: Pergamon.

Niaura, R.S., Rohsenow, D.J., Binkoff, J.A., Monti, P.M., Pedraza, M. & Abrams, D.B. (1988). The relevance of cue reactivity to understanding alcohol and smoking relapse. *Journal of Abnormal Psychology*, **97**, 133–152.

O'Malley, S.S., Jaffe, A.J., Chang, G., Schottenfeld, R.S., Meyer, R.E. & Rounsaville, B. (1992). Naltrexone and coping skills therapy for alcohol dependence. *Archives of General Psychiaty*, **49**, 881–887.

Pead, J., Greeley, J., Ritter, A., Murray, T., Felstead, B., Mattick, R. & Heather, N. (1993). A clinical trial of cue exposure combined with cognitive-behavioral treatment for alcohol dependence. Presented at the 55th Meeting of the College on Problems of Drug Dependence, Toronto, June.

Pickens, R., Bigelow, G. & Griffiths, R. (1973). An experimental approach to treating chronic alcoholism: a case study and one-year follow-up. *Behaviour Research and Therapy*, **11**, 321–325.

Pomerleau, O.F. (1981). Underlying mechanisms in substance abuse: examples from research on smoking. *Addictive Behaviors*, **6**, 187–196.

Rankin, H.J. (1982). Cue exposure and response prevention in South London. In P. Nathan and W. Hay (Eds), *Case Studies in the Behavioral Modification of Alcoholism*, pp. 227–248. New York: Plenum Press.

Rankin, H., Hodgson, R. & Stockwell, T. (1983). Cue exposure and response prevention with alcoholics: a controlled trial. *Behaviour Research and Therapy*, **21**, 435–446.

Rohsenow, D.J., Monti, P.M., Rubonis, A.V., Goddard, P.G., Niaura, R.S., Abrams, D.B., Sirota, A.B. & Colby, S. (1989). Alcohol cue reactivity during detoxification. In D.J. Rohsenow (Chair), "Recent advances in cue reactivity research in the addictions." Symposium presented at the Annual Meeting of the Association for Advancement of Behavior Therapy, Washington, DC.

Rohsenow, D.J., Niaura, R.S., Childress, A.R., Abrams, D.B. & Monti, P.M. (1990). Cue reactivity in addictive behaviors: theoretical and treatment implications. *International Journal of the Addictions*, **25**, 957–993.

Rohsenow, D.J., Monti, P.M., Abrams, D.B., Rubonis, A.V., Niaura, R.S., Sirota, A.D. & Colby, S.M. (1992). Cue elicited urge to drink and salivation in alcoholics: relationship to individual differences. *Advances in Behaviour Research and Therapy*, **14**, 195–210.

Rohsenow, D.J., Monti, P.M., Rubonis, A.V., Sirota, A.D., Niaura, R.S., Colby, S.M., Wunschel, S.M. & Abrams, D.B. (1994). Cue reactivity as a predictor of drinking among male alcoholics. *Journal of Consulting and Clinical Psychology*, **62**, 620–626.

Rubonis, A.V., Colby, S.M., Monti, P.M., Rohsenow, D.J., Gulliver, S.B. & Sirota,

A.D. (1994). Alcohol cue reactivity and mood induction in male and female alcoholics. *Journal of Studies on Alcohol*, **55**, 487–494.

Sartory, G., Rachman, S. & Grey, S.J. (1982). Return of fear: the role of rehearsal. *Behaviour Research and Therapy*, **20**, 123–133.

Sayette, M.A., Monti, P.M., Rohsenow, D.J., Gulliver, S.B., Colby, S.M., Sirota, A.D., Niaura, R.S. and Abrams, D.B. (1995). The effects of cue exposure on reaction time in male alcoholics. *Journal of Studies on Alcohol*, in press.

Siegal, S. (1979). The role of conditioning in drug tolerance and addiction. In J.D. Keehn (Ed.), *Psychopathology in Animals: Research and Clinical Applications*. New York: Academic Press.

Staiger, P.K. & White, J.M. (1991). Cue reactivity in alcohol abusers: stimulus specificity and extinction of the responses. *Addictive Behaviors*, **16**, 211–221.

Staiger, P.K., Greeley, J., Pead, J. & Horne, D. (1993). Cue exposure with alcohol dependents: findings from a controlled trial and one year follow-up study. In P.M. Monti (Chair), "Cue exposure and alcohol treatment: where do we stand?" Symposium conducted at the Sixth International Conference on Treatment of Addictive Behaviors, Santa Fe, NM, January.

Stasiewicz, P.R. & Maisto, S.A. (1993). Two-factor avoidance theory: the role of negative affect in the maintenance of substance use and substance use disorder. *Behavior Therapy*, **24**, 337–356.

Stewart, J., de Wit, H. & Eikelboom, R. (1984). The role of unconditioned and conditioned drug effects in the self-administration of opiates and stimulants. *Psychological Review*, **91**, 251–268.

Tiffany, S.T. (1990). A cognitive model of drug urges and drug-use behavior: the role of automatic and nonautomatic processes. *Psychological Review*, **97**, 147–168.

Twentyman, C.T., Greenwald, D.P., Greenwald, M.A., Kloss, J.D., Kovaleski, M.E. & Zibung-Hoffman, P. (1982). An assessment of social skill deficits in alcoholics. *Behavioral Assessment*, **4**, 317–326.

Wardle, J. (1990). Conditioning processes and cue exposure in the modification of excessive eating. *Addictive Behaviors*, **15**, 387–393.

Wilson, G.T. (1981). Expectations and substance abuse: does basic research benefit clinical assessment and therapy? *Addictive Behaviors*, **6**, 221–231.

CHAPTER 9

Cue exposure treatment in opiate and cocaine dependence

Sharon Dawe* and Jane H. Powell⁺

Given the clearly demonstrated benefits of exposure-based techniques in the treatment of previously intractable problems such as obsessive compulsive disorder and phobias (e.g. Marks, 1987) it is not surprising that researchers and clinicians working with substance misusers have advocated the use of cue exposure in addictive behaviours. Such optimism is not unfounded. Dating from the seminal work of Wikler, a substantial body of empirical research has provided strong evidence for a conditioning model of addiction (see Wikler, 1975, 1980, for reviews).

With respect to opiate addiction, both drug-like and drug-opposite conditioned responses have been demonstrated experimentally with human opiate addicts (O'Brien et al., 1974, 1975; Wikler, 1975, 1980). Withdrawal-like responses have been demonstrated in opiate addicts (or detoxified opiate addicts) in a number of studies (see O'Brien et al., 1992, for a review). For example, Teasdale (1973) found that detoxified opiate addicts had an increase in self-reported withdrawal symptoms and ratings of tension and confusion when exposed to drug-related slides. In a similar setting, Powell, Bradley & Gray (1992) also found an increase in self-reported withdrawal symptoms and craving using both opiate-related slides and more potent cues such as needles and syringes, and simulated heroin powder. Physiological responses such as increases in heart rate and galvanic skin response consistent with opiate withdrawal have been reported when opiate addicts in the final stages of methadone detoxification were exposed to a videotape depicting heroin preparation and use (Sideroff & Jarvik, 1980).

---

*University of New South Wales, Sydney, Australia, and ⁺University of London, UK.

Addictive Behaviour: Cue Exposure Theory and Practice.
Edited by D.C. Drummond, S.T. Tiffany, S. Glautier and B. Remington.
© 1995 John Wiley & Sons Ltd.

Conversely, conditioned drug-like responses have been demonstrated in controlled laboratory settings when opiates have been available. Heroin addicts who were allowed to self-inject in a laboratory setting exhibited drug-like subjective and physiological responses (O'Brien et al., 1975). Similarly, a 'cook-up' procedure produced opiate-like responses in ex-heroin addicts when they self-administered opiates under naltrexone blockade (see O'Brien et al., 1992). Extending this procedure to a naturalistic setting, Powell (1990) found that opiate addicts maintained on injectable methadone experienced a reduction in self-reported withdrawal symptoms and an increase in positive mood when they began their preparation for self-injection in their own home, an environment strongly associated with injection as they had been maintained on injectable methadone for an average of 10 months. It is possible that one factor influencing the direction of conditioned responding is the individual's expectation of the actual possibility that the substance in question will be administered. Data relevant to this point were reported by Glautier, Drummond & Remington (1992). When subjects received instructions that they were going to drink alcohol as part of the experiment they showed anticipatory alcohol-like responses.

Although less systematically investigated, laboratory studies have found that cocaine-related cues reliably elicit conditioned responses. Ehrman et al. (1992), comparing responsivity to cocaine-related cues, opiate-related cues and neutral cues in cocaine addicts, reported that cocaine addicts showed significantly greater response to the cocaine-related cues than to opiate-related or neutral stimuli. While the physiological responses were consistent with the stimulant effect of cocaine, i.e. increases in heart rate, skin resistance and skin temperature, subjects reported a significant increase in withdrawal symptoms and craving and did not consistently report an increase in cocaine high. Thus, while these findings are consistent with a conditioning model of addiction, it would appear that both conditioned drug-like and conditioned drug-opposite responses were observed. However, Kranzler & Bauer (1992) found that subjects exposed to cocaine-associated stimuli and to neutral stimuli reported an increase in desire for cocaine and an increase in 'euphoria'. This index was derived from a scale comprising ratings of each of the following symptoms: high, tight chest, rush/thrill, sweating, and pounding heart. However, it is relevant to note that these symptoms may be related to nonspecific arousal symptoms rather than to specific drug-like symptoms. Unlike Ehrman et al.'s (1992) study there was no effect of exposure to cocaine-associated stimuli on withdrawal.

It is difficult to account for the differences in responsivity between various studies. It is likely that other factors such as the magnitude of the reinforcement associated with the direct drug effect (e.g. Foltin & Fischman, 1992) and the onset effect of the drug (see de Wit, Bodker & Ambre, 1992) also influence the direction of the conditioned response.

Regardless of whether the direction of the conditioned response is determined by the accessibility of the substance in question, the magnitude of the unconditioned effect or by the rapidity of the drug effect, the premise that conditioned responses are implicated in the relapse process is still strongly favoured. A former addict returning to an environment in which he or she had used drugs may encounter numerous external cues; the environment itself, abandoned needles and syringes, and individuals with whom the former addict had associated may all have become conditioned stimuli (CS) which will elicit conditioned responses (CRs). The experience of CRs may be one of the many factors that influence an individual to engage in drug-seeking behaviour, and ultimately, drug use. An individual experiencing conditioned withdrawal-like responses would be in an aversive physical and emotional state that would be alleviated, i.e. negatively reinforced, by the administration of drugs. Alternatively, conditioned drug-like responses might generate an appetitive motivational state via 'priming', increasing the likelihood that the former addict will take steps to administer the previously abused drug or a drug with similar stimulus properties (Stewart, de Wit & Eikelboom, 1984).

There are now several studies in which cue exposure techniques have been used in the treatment of opiate addiction. These studies have, in some respects, been promising, particularly in relation to the impact of the treatment on process variables such as craving and cue reactivity. For instance, Childress et al. (1987) found a significant reduction in craving and withdrawal symptoms to drug-related cues, in abstinent opiate and cocaine users, following 20 1 hour long cue exposure sessions. In case reports of two detoxified heroin addicts and one solvent abuser, Bradley & Moorey (1988) reported a decrease in craving within the actual sessions, i.e. within-session habituation, and a decline in overall levels of craving across sessions, i.e. between-session habituation. In the first controlled trial of cue exposure (Powell, Bradley & Gray, 1992) recently detoxified opiate addicts received two sessions of either cue exposure or cue exposure with cognitive aversion or a control no-treatment condition. Subjects receiving both the cue exposure and cue exposure with cognitive aversion showed a significant decrease in craving and self-reported withdrawal symptoms to probe stimuli presented before and after the cue exposure treatment, across a 1 week period. It is notable that the control subjects, tested at the same time points as the two treatment groups, showed no such reductions.

On the basis of these promising results a larger clinical trial, using similar treatment methodology to that developed in this pilot study, was conducted by Dawe et al. (1993). In this trial, recently detoxified opiate addicts were allocated randomly to cue exposure or control conditions. Cue exposure subjects received a minimum of six cue exposure sessions and, after hospital discharge, all subjects were followed up at about 6 weeks and again at 6 months. Contrary to Powell at al.'s (1992) findings, both control subjects and cue exposure subjects were found to show a significant decrease on measures of cue reactivity when reassessed at the same time points, i.e. 3 weeks from an initial assessment for the control subjects and following at least six sessions of cue exposure for the experimental subjects. In attempting to account for the decline in cue reactivity in the control group, Dawe et al. (1993) suggested that subjects in both groups may have received sufficient informal or unstructured cue exposure in the standard hospital treatment program. Standard treatment included group discussion of issues relating to drug use and training in relapse prevention. In addition, subjects were able to return to their own homes on weekend and day leave, arguably allowing for extinction to environmental drug cues to occur. It may therefore be argued that a time- and therapist-intensive structured cue exposure treatment of the kind described is not necessary to obtain extinction of conditioned responses in opiate addicts who are already receiving a comprehensive treatment package.

On the basis of this one controlled treatment trial it would appear that initially optimistic findings from early studies were not borne out when cue exposure was rigorously evaluated in terms of its effect on relapse. However, it would be premature to suggest, on the basis of a negative result from the only completed controlled trial, that cue exposure cannot confer any additional benefit over and above a well-structured treatment program. Indeed, it is the present authors' view that cue exposure treatment may well be appropriate for a subset of opiate addicts. There may be factors in the design of the treatment protocol or the selection of appropriate subjects that are critical in determining the effectiveness of cue exposure. The next section of this chapter examines a range of such factors and emphasizes the importance of considering these in relation both to clinical practice and future research.

Given the current uncertainty concerning the usefulness of cue exposure in the treatment of opiate and cocaine addiction, it is important to optimize its clinical potential by paying heed to the widest possible range of theoretically and empirically derived considerations in designing a treatment protocol. Theoretical design factors are derived from a detailed scrutiny of the mechanisms postulated to underlie the treatment, and in the case of cue exposure fall into two main groups: those relating to classical conditioning on the one hand, and those relating to cognitive factors on the other. Empirical considerations include factors relating to the palatability, viability and relevance of the treatment to the population of addicts presenting for help.

THEORETICAL DESIGN CONSIDERATIONS

Classical Conditioning Mechanisms

The basic mechanisms of classical conditioning, particularly as they apply to drug addiction, have already been described in detail in earlier chapters. One rationale for the cue exposure approach is the interpretation that the subjective and physiological reactions shown by addicts during exposure to drug-related stimuli are CRs which have been established through repeated pairings of drug-induced unconditioned responses (URs) (drug-positive or withdrawal-like) with stimuli regularly present in the environment at the time of onset of these responses.

According to classical conditioning theory, extinction of these CRs can be achieved through repeated unreinforced exposure to the CS, the CR becoming progressively weaker in terms of both intensity and duration across successive exposures. When demonstrated in the animal laboratory, this phenomenon of between-session habituation is usually secondary to a process of within-session habituation in which, during individual exposure trials, the CR rises to peak intensity before gradually reducing across the remainder of the exposure. There is evidence to suggest that if exposure is terminated whilst the CR is at, or close to, its peak intensity then sensitization may be observed (Groves & Thompson, 1970), implying that the CR would become more pronounced in a subsequent exposure to the CS.

In clinical applications of cue exposure with anxiety disorders, it has been reported by Foa (1979) that the treatment was effective in reducing anxiety levels across sessions only if within-session habituation was achieved. Although the necessity for this has not been systematically investigated within addiction research, comparisons of different protocols which have been employed do suggest that it is a relevant factor. Thus, for instance, Childress, McLellan & O'Brien (1986) employed fixed duration stimulus presentations of 10 minutes each with methadone-maintained addicts, three times weekly and for a total of 35 sessions. Across the group as a whole, however, an elevation of the craving response was apparent across at least the first 10 sessions, with between-session habituation being seen thereafter. By contrast, in a later study of cue exposure with abstinent opiate and cocaine users (Childress et al., 1987), in which extinction sessions were 1 hour each, conditioned craving and conditioned withdrawal were substantially reduced within the first 10 sessions. In studies by Powell, Bradley & Gray (1992) and Dawe et al. (1993), where stimulus presentations were terminated only when within-session habituation of craving had occurred, there was marked between-session habituation across only two to five sessions.

Another issue highly relevant to treatment is the selection of stimuli which are personally relevant to the individual addict. The premise of the classical conditioning analysis is that drug-positive and/or withdrawal symptoms become CRs via a process of association with specific contextual stimuli. If treatment is to be effective in promoting extinction of such CRs, then exposure clearly should be to stimuli which have had the opportunity to become CSs for the particular individual being treated. Clinically this has been stressed by O'Brien's research group on the basis of experience in early studies conducted in their laboratory. In practice, although certain stimuli may be excluded as irrelevant to an individual on the basis of interview information (e.g. syringes may not have become CRs for an addict who uses a different route of ingestion and avoids contact with injectors), it may be necessary to test the relevance of other stimuli by presenting them to the addict and observing responses to them. Using such an empirical approach, Dawe et al. (1993) were able to concentrate with individual addicts on just those stimuli from the available repertoire which were effective in eliciting a response. It is also possible that this individualized approach to exposure facilitated the rapid extinction found in this study, where the average total duration of cue exposure was just under 5 hours (six or seven sessions).

Where an individual fails to show quantifiable responses to drug cues at their initial presentation it is clearly difficult to ascertain whether exposure is achieving any immediate effects and a decision about when to terminate treatment will have to be made on other grounds. It should be stressed, however, that the most important test of any form of cue exposure treatment is not the observable impact on cue reactivity but rather its impact on subsequent drug use. Since few outcome studies have thus far been conducted, it remains logically possible that a fixed number of cue exposure sessions will be effective in eliminating CRs which are, for various reasons, not accessible to measurement during treatment.

Related to the issue of relevant treatment stimuli is that of generalization of treatment effects. Given the vast number of contextual cues which have regularly been associated with symptoms of drug use or withdrawal, it is obviously impossible to attempt the extinction of responses to each and every CS. However, it is reasonable to assume from classical conditioning theory that there will be generalization of habituation achieved in relation to one CS to other CSs which bear some resemblance to it. It may be constructive therefore to select for exposure treatment those stimuli which are likely to be of most widespread occurrence in the addict's learning history, for example the drug-using equipment itself, or specific geographical locations of drug use. Other stimuli which co-occur with these key stimuli, but are less frequently present or less salient, are theoretically likely to accrue some benefit of exposure treatment by generalization. Consistent with this view, Powell, Bradley & Gray (1992) demonstrated a reduction in craving to stimuli which were not themselves incorporated into an exposure treatment program.

Within this framework, the range of cues which are theoretically potent range from simple pictorial stimuli to actual drug ingestion under conditions of pharmacological blockade (O'Brien et al, 1979). Since the real-life test of cue exposure treatment lies in the ability to resist the temptation to use when faced with a situation in which drugs are actually available, there is a strong case for emphasizing the importance of including situations approximating as closely as possible to this in the exposure treatment. A number of difficulties have, however, emerged in attempts to achieve this. O'Brien's group reported that the self-administration of opiates under blockade, and likewise the injection of an inert substance, proved highly aversive to subjects, resulting in a high drop-out rate. Dawe et al. (1993) included *in vivo* exposure to drug-using locations in their treatment program, with therapists accompanying detoxified addicts on visits to these places in order to monitor their reactions and help them to wait for habituation of any craving to occur (Groves & Thompson, 1970). In practice, however, there were occasions when it was impossible to remain in the presence of drug cues for sufficient time to allow a diminution in craving that was consistent with the requirement of within-session habituation. Within the real environment the most potent cue observed was the offer of heroin by a known drug dealer. Practical and safety considerations make it impossible to remain in the presence of this highly salient cue. However, removing the cue, or moving away from it, may be seen as removing the stimulus at a point when the response is maximal thereby allowing for the possibility of sensitization to occur. Whilst it may theoretically be preferable to send subjects out on such visits unaccompanied, this also carries with it the risk that the temptation to use might be too strong to be resisted, a consideration which is likely to generate opposition from other professionals involved in an addict's treatment. Nevertheless, given that this will be the situation to which the addict returns after discharge from treatment, there is a strong case for arguing that cue exposure treatment should include carefully selected *in vivo* exposure.

Safer, and of considerable demonstrated potency in eliciting craving in opiate addicts, is the use of self-generated imagery (Dawe et al., 1993). This has been explored in more depth in the cue exposure treatment of alcoholism and certainly deserves more investigation with opiate addicts. Whilst exposure to imagined situations still falls qualitatively short of exposure to real-life situations, in that imaginal cues do not signal genuine and immediate drug availability, they may approximate quite closely to the situation in which the addict experiences a desire for drugs but has to then go to some lengths to procure them. Furthermore, the use of imagery cues in other contexts has proved powerful in eliciting powerful and realistic affective reactions (e.g. Kozak, Foa & Steketee, 1988).

Cognitive Mechanisms

Another possible mechanism influencing the magnitude of responses to drug-related cues is essentially cognitive in nature: the elicitation of a set of outcome expectancies concerning the likelihood and desirability of possible drug effects. Social learning theory analyses applied to the understanding of addiction (e.g. Marlatt & Gordon, 1985) suggest that the more powerful an individual expects drugs to be in producing subjectively desirable effects, and the fewer alternative strategies he/she perceives for achieving these, then the stronger will be the desire to seek out and use drugs. If craving is experienced as the affective concomitant of positive outcome expectancies, then the cognitive dimension may be critical during cue exposure itself.

There is some evidence to support an association between positive outcome expectancies for substance use and both desire for and actual use of drugs in the fields of alcoholism (Brown, 1985) and opiate addiction (Powell et al., 1993). Of particular interest in the context of the substrate to craving during cue exposure, Cooney et al. (1987) found an increase in self-rated positive outcome expectancies for alcohol use immediately following exposure to alcohol-related cues. Furthermore, there was a significant correlation between the level of positive expectancies and the magnitude of self-reported desire to drink. Relatedly, with opiate addicts, Bradley & Moorey (1988) found that verbal distractions during cue exposure with opiate addicts (e.g. oral repetition of a nursery rhyme) resulted in a rapid reduction in self-reported craving. There was, however, no sustained benefit of this quickly achieved reduction in craving: in subsequent sessions craving at the original level was reinstated.

Findings such as these do at least highlight the importance of ensuring that addicts' attention is appropriately focused during cue exposure treatment. Foa & Kozak (1986) stress the need to ensure that anxious patients undergoing cue exposure are not cognitively distracting themselves from salient stimuli, and it would sensible to adopt a similar stance in applying the approach to opiate addicts. It may also be fruitful to exploit the potential influence of cognitive factors by actively teaching individuals to generate aversive thoughts or imagery which may counteract positive expectancies elicited by drug-related stimuli and thus help to reduce the level of craving experienced. In a small controlled study, Powell, Bradley & Gray (1992) evaluated the effect of combining cue exposure with instructions to think about and verbalize aversive aspects of drug use. Across two such exposure sessions, subjects receiving the combined treatment showed reductions in craving which were equivalent to, but no greater than, those shown by subjects receiving cue exposure alone.

Although this finding suggests that formalized instructions to generate negative outcome expectancies did not promote speedier or greater reductions in craving, it was noted anecdotally that subjects in the cue exposure alone group did spontaneously report aversive thoughts taking the place of positive expectancies in parallel with reductions in craving. It remains possible, then, that for individual subjects explicit encouragement to use cognitive strategies to reduce craving may be of benefit. Further, it is also possible that the application of such strategies in a real-world high-risk situation in which drugs are readily available may be used to achieve a rapid reduction of craving to a more controllable level.

Finally, there may be an interaction between the conditioned response elicited by the drug cue and actual availability of the drug for self-administration. As discussed above, there are indications that drug-like conditioned responses may be elicited in settings when the subject knows that he/she has access to the drug. Traditionally, cue exposure treatment has not involved the presence of the actual drug but simply cues associated with its use, to which the predominant response elicited is withdrawal-like. When simulated heroin has been used (e.g. Dawe et al., 1993) the subject has been aware that the substance is inert. It has been suggested (Powell, 1990) that in the laboratory setting such cues may in fact signal drug *non*-availability, hence triggering conditioned withdrawal instead of a conditioned drug-like reaction. Thus, it can be argued that laboratory-based cue exposure treatment will preferentially extinguish conditioned withdrawal responses, but that when the subject returns to an environment previously associated with drug use, the real possibility of administration may result in the elicitation of conditioned drug-like responses. While this is speculative and requires empirical validation, it is possible that the efficacy of cue exposure treatment may be enhanced if subjects believed that it was actually possible to use their drug of choice. While ethical and legal considerations may limit the use of the actual drug when the subject's preferred drug is illicit, it may be that these additional considerations could first be evaluated in populations whose problem substance is not illegal, i.e. alcohol or cigarettes.

EMPIRICAL CONSIDERATIONS

Individuals who present for treatment for cocaine or opiate dependence bring with them a range of psychosocial problems, many that can be seen to be directly related to drug use such as involvement in criminal activity, unemployment, or a social network of drug users; some that may be predisposing factors that led to drug use such as a history of childhood physical or sexual abuse. In addition many substance misusers have other concurrent psychiatric disorders or concurrent alcohol dependence problems that have been associated with poorer outcome (e.g. Carroll et al., 1993). Given such a complex social and psychological profile it would be unlikely that any single treatment offered over a relatively short period of time would have sufficient impact in this population. Cue exposure is no exception. Thus, the question then becomes whether cue exposure, in conjunction with other treatment methods and interventions, confers some additional benefit over the standard treatment offered. In the study by Dawe et al. (1993) this was not the case. However, is may be that there is a subgroup of addicts for whom cue exposure may be a more beneficial treatment. Typically, one-thid of subjects in cue reactivity studies do not report increases in subjective measures of desire or craving (e.g. Powell, Bradley & Gray, 1993; McLellan et al., 1986). Whether cue exposure is a treatment that is more appropriate for individuals who have a reaction to drug-related cues remains an empirical question, but one that warrants further investigation.

CONCLUSION

Cue exposure has been viewed as a promising treatment by both researchers and clinicians for individuals with addictive behaviour problems (e.g. Heather & Bradley, 1990; Hodgson, 1991). There is now a substantial body of evidence to support a conditioning model of addiction, and preliminary case reports and uncontrolled treatment trials suggest that cue exposure may indeed hold promise for those involved in the difficult business of treating opiate and cocaine abusers. However, in the only randomized controlled trial of cue exposure with opiate addicts so far conducted (Dawe et al., 1993), cue exposure did not confer any additional benefit over and above a standard (albeit comprehensive) inpatient treatment programme. Despite this finding, it is the present authors' view that it would be premature to dismiss cue exposure as a useful treatment option. Instead, further research should focus on the components of cue exposure that may be effective in facilitating behaviour change. Drawing from the extensive findings from the anxiety literature, we argue that cue exposure sessions should involve exposure to graded cues that are individually tailored to the addict, that cue-elicited responses should return to a baseline level before the introduction of another cue and that treatment should focus on the cue and not incorporate elements that may serve to distract the addict. Further, whenever practicable, treatment should involve an *in vivo* component that will allow for a process of habituation and, for some individuals, an opportunity for exposure to drug cues in an environment in which drug use is an option.

However, it is unlikely that cue exposure as a treatment for opiate or cocaine abuse alone will ever produce the significant treatment gains found in the anxiety literature. Opiate and cocaine use is associated with a range of social and psychological problems that will need to be addressed if the individual is to have a reasonable chance of remaining drug free after treatment.

REFERENCES

Bradley, B.P. & Moorey, S. (1988). Extinction of craving during exposure to drug-related cues: three single case reports. *Behavioural Psychotherapy*, **16**, 45–56.

Brown, S.A. (1985). Reinforcement expectancies and alcoholism treatment outcome after a one-year follow-up. *Journal of Studies on Alcohol*, **46**, 304–308.

Carroll, K.M., Power, M.D., Bryant, K.J. & Rounsaville, B.J. (1993). One year follow-up status of treatment seeking cocaine abusers: psychopathology and dependence severity as predictors of outcome. *Journal of Nervous and Mental Disease*, **181**, 71–79.

Childress, A.R., McLellan, A.T. & O'Brien, C.P. (1986). Role of conditioning factors in the development of drug dependence. *Psychiatric Clinics of North America*, **9**, 413–425.

Childress, A.R., McLellan, A.T., Ehrman, R.N. & O'Brien, C.P. (1987). Extinction of conditioned responses in abstinent cocaine or opioid users. In *Problems of Drug Dependence*, NIDA Research Monograph No. 76, pp. 137–144. Washington DC: US Government Printing Office.

Cooney, N.L., Gillespie, R.A., Baker, L.H. & Kaplan, R.F. (1987). Cognitive changes after alcohol cue exposure. *Journal of Consulting and Clinical Psychology*, **55**, 150–155.

Dawe, S., Powell, J.H., Richards, D., Gossop, M., Marks, I., Strang, J. & Gray, J.A. (1993). Does post-withdrawal cue exposure influence outcome in opiate addiction: a controlled trial. *Addiction*, **88**, 1227–1239.

de Wit, H., Bodker, B.K. & Ambre, J. (1992). Rate of increase of plasma drug level influences subjective response in humans. *Psychopharmacology*, **107**, 352–358.

Ehrman, R.M., Robbins, S.J., Childress, A.R. & O'Brien, C.P. (1992). Conditioned responses to cocaine-related stimuli in cocaine abuse patients. *Psychopharmacology*, **107**, 523–529.

Foa, E.B. (1979). Failure in treating obsessive-compulsives. *Behaviour Research and Therapy*, **17**, 169–176.

Foa, E.B. & Kozak, M.J. (1986). Emotional processing of fear: exposure to corrective information. *Psychological Bulletin*, **99**, 20–35.

Foltin, R.W. & Fischman, M.W. (1992). Self-administration of cocaine by humans: choice between smoked and intravenous cocaine. *Journal of Pharmacology and Experimental Therapeutics*, **261**, 841–849.

Glautier, S., Drummond, D.C. & Remington, R. (1992). Different drink cues elicit different physiological responses in non-dependent drinkers. *Psychopharmacology*, **106**, 550–554.

Groves, P.M. & Thompson, R.F. (1970). Habituation: a dual-process theory *Psychological Review*, **77**, 419–450.

Heather, N. & Bradley, B. (1990). Cue exposure as a practical treatment for addictive disorders: why are we waiting? *Addictive Behaviors*, **15**, 335–337.

Hodgson, R. (1991). Substance misuse. *Behavioral Psychotherapy*, **90**, 80–87.

Kozak, M.J., Foa, E.B. & Steketee, G. (1988). Process and outcome of exposure treatment with obsessive-compulsives: physiological indicators of emotional processing. *Behavior Therapy*, **19**, 157–169.

Kranzler, H.R. & Bauer, L.O. (1992). Bromocriptine and cocaine cue reactivity in cocaine-dependent patients. *British Journal of Addiction*, **87**, 1537–1548.

Marks, I.M. (1987). Behavioural and drug treatments of phobic and obsessive compulsive disorders. *Psychotherapy and Psychosomatics*, **46**, 35–44.

Marlatt, G.A. & Gordon, J.R. (1985). *Relapse Prevention Techniques: Maintenance Strategies in the Treatment of Addictive Behaviours*. New York: Guilford Press.

McLellan, A.T., Childress, A.R., Ehrman, R., O'Brien, C.P. & Pashko, S. (1986). Extinguishing conditioned responses during opiate dependence treatment: turning laboratory findings into clinical procedures. *Journal of Substance Abuse Treatment*, **3**, 33–40.

O'Brien, C.P., Chaddock, B., Woody, B. & Greenstein, R. (1974). Systematic extinction of narcotic drug use using narcotic antagonists. *Psychosomatic Medicine*, **36**, 458.

O'Brien, C.P., O'Brien, T.J., Mintz, J. & Brady, J.P. (1975). Conditioning of narcotic abstinence syndrome in human subjects. *Drug and Alcohol Dependence*, **1**, 115–123.

O'Brien, C.P., Greenstein, R., Ternes, J., McLellan, A.T. & Grabowski, J. (1979). Unreinforced self-injections: effects on rituals and outcome in heroin addicts. In L.S. Harris (Ed.), *Proceedings of the 41st Annual Scientific Meeting of the Committee on Problems of Drug Abuse*, NIDA Research Monograph No. 27, pp. 265–381. Washington DC: US Government Printing Office.

O'Brien, C.P., Childress, A.R., McLellan, A.T. & Ehrman, R. (1992). A learning model of addiction. In C.P. O'Brien, C.P. & J.H. Jaffe (Eds), *Addictive States,* Vol. 70, Association for Research in Nervous and Mental Disease. New York: Raven Press.

Powell (1990). Cue exposure in opiate addiction: effects and mechanisms. PhD Thesis, University of London.

Powell, J.H., Bradley, B. & Gray, J.A. (1992). Subjective craving for opiates: evaluation of a cue exposure protocol for use with detoxified opiate addicts. *British Journal of Clinical Psychology,* **32**, 39–53.

Powell, J., Dawe, S., Richards, D., Gossop, M., Marks, I., Strang, J. & Gray, J.A. (1993). Can opiate addicts tell us about their relapse risk? Subjective predictors of clinical prognosis. *Addictive Behaviors,* **18**, 473–490.

Sideroff, S. & Jarvik, M.E. (1980). Conditioned responses to a video showing heroin-related stimuli. *International Journal of the Addictions,* **15**, 529–536.

Stewart, J., de Wit, H. & Eikelboom, R. (1984). Role of unconditioned and conditioned drug effects in the self-administration of opiates and stimulants. *Psychological Review,* **91**, 251–268.

Teasdale, J.D. (1973). Conditioned abstinence in narcotic addicts. *International Journal of the Addictions,* **8**, 273–292.

Wikler, A. (1975). Opioid antagonists and deconditioning in addiction treatment. In H. Bostrom, T. Larsson & N. Ljungstedt (Eds), *Drug Dependence—Treatment and Treatment Evaluation.* Stockholm: Almqvist and Wiskell International.

Wikler, A. (1980). *Opioid Dependence: Mechanisms and Treatment,* New York: Plenum Press.

CHAPTER 10   Cue exposure treatment in nicotine dependence

Thomas H. Brandon,* Thomas M. Piasecki,† Edward P. Quinn* and Timothy B. Baker†

Tobacco smoking, like other substance abuse, is a behavior that is notoriously resistant to long-term change. Although treatments now exist that can reliably produce short-term cessation in the great majority of motivated smokers (e.g. Hall et al., 1984; Zelman et al., 1992), no treatment consistently produces year-long abstinence rates that exceed 50%. In recent years researchers have searched for new interventions with potential for improving the long-term outcome of smoking cessation treatments. One such technique is cue exposure therapy, which was originally based on the premise that certain stimuli, through their association with nicotine intake, become classically conditioned stimuli (CSs) that elicit conditioned responses (CRs; e.g. urges to smoke or activation of drug motivational systems). These same stimuli may also serve as discriminative stimuli (SD) that signal the availability of positive or negative reinforcement through smoking. In these ways, smoking-related stimuli might motivate smoking, even long after initial cessation. By exposing smokers to these stimuli in the absence of nicotine intake, the associative links should be altered or extinguished. (See Glautier & Remington, Chapter 2 and Tiffany, Chapters 3 and 7 for reviews of associative and non-associative theories related to cue exposure effects.)

EXISTING RESEARCH

Cue Reactivity

To test for a causal relationship between smoking-related stimuli and motivation to smoke (if not actual relapse) researchers have turned to

---

*State University of New York at Binghamton, New York and †University of Wisconsin-Madison, Wisconsin, USA

Addictive Behaviour: Cue Exposure Theory and Practice.
Edited by D.C. Drummond, S.T. Tiffany, S. Glautier and B. Remington.

laboratory-controlled cue reactivity experiments. These studies examine smokers' responses (self-report, physiological, and/or behavioral) to smoking-related and neutral cues. Differential responding to smoking-related cues is presumed to reflect a history of classical conditioning. This is merely a presumption because, unlike drug conditioning research with infra-human subjects, the experimenter has had no control over the conditioning trials. In only one single-subject study has a researcher attempted to classically condition arbitrary stimuli to cigarette smoke intake (Payne, Etscheidt & Corrigan, 1990). After 20 conditioning trials, the subject evidenced a 23% greater puff duration when exposed to the CS compared to stimuli previously paired with mock smoking. Physiological responses, however, not did not show a clear conditioning effect.

Several studies have now shown that exposure to smoking-related cues elicits greater reactivity across a number of response domains than does exposure to neutral cues. Cues used include viewing or holding a cigarette (Herman, 1974; Sayette & Hufford, 1993), live or videotaped smoking by others (Rickard-Figueroa & Zeichner, 1985; Surawy, Stepney & Cox, 1985), smoking-related imagery (Tiffany & Hakenewerth, 1991), and combinations of these (Niaura et al., 1992). In addition, a number of researchers have extended the cue reactivity paradigm to include not only environmental cues, but also interoceptive cues—negative affect in particular. Negative affect has been induced by imagery (Tiffany & Drobes, 1990), uncontrollable noise blasts (Payne et al., 1991), and false feedback on an intelligence test (Brandon, Wetter & Baker, 1994).

Although all of these studies found evidence of cue reactivity, they differ in terms of which response domains showed the reactivity. Of the studies that assessed self-reported urge or desire to smoke, all but one (Niaura et al., 1992) found that smoking-related cues increased such ratings. Cardiovascular measures (blood pressure, heart rate) also have tended to show cue reactivity effects, though not as consistently as have urge ratings. Recently, Sayette & Hufford (1994) also found that simple reaction time to a tone simulus increased during cue exposure. Finally a few studies have allowed subjects to smoke following cue exposure, and have measured 'smoking topography' variables assumed to reflect motivation to smoke. Herman (1974) found that exposure to a high salience cue (the sight of cigarettes) was associated with a shorter latency to smoke and a greater number of cigarettes smoked compared to a low salience cue, especially among lighter smokers. Payne and his colleagues (1991) also found that smoking-related cues led to a shorter latency to smoke, as well as a greater total amount of time spent inhaling. They additionally found that negative affect induction produced an increase in other topography measures. Surawy, Stepney & Cox (1985) reported that for a subset of smokers ('stimulant' smokers), cue exposure led to decreased latency to smoke and increased number of cigarettes smoked. However, two studies failed to find exposure effects on self-administration measures, including latency to smoke (Brandon, Wetter & Baker, 1994; Niaura et al., 1992). Moreover, these same two studies, as well as Tiffany & Hakenewerth (1991), explicitly noted a pattern of low correlations across the different response modes (urge self-report, physiological, and behavioral), which challenges the assumption that the responses all reflect a common underlying motivation to smoke.

The relation between cue reactivity and relapse following treatment was examined in a study by Abrams and his colleagues (Abrams et al., 1988, Study 2). At the 6 month follow-up, subjects were dichotomized into relapsers and abstainers and these two groups were compared on pre- and post-treatment cue reactivity. Relapsers were found to have had greater heart rate reactivity following the pre-treatment cue exposure (watching a confederate smoke), and they also had reported greater anxiety. No group differences were found on galvanic skin conductance or urge ratings. However, a second analysis of the data using an increased sample size found that post-treatment, rather than pre-treatment heart rate reactivity predicted 6 month outcome (Niaura et al.,1989).

In summary, cue reactivity research has shown that smokers exhibit reactivity to cues associated with smoking (including negative affect) compared to neutral cues, although the nature of the response differs across studies. This parallels findings with alcohol, opiates, and cocaine. It is not clear that the cue reactivity measured in these studies truly reflects a classically conditioned response—e.g. it might reflect mental work that could have innumerable bases: appraisal of the stimulus, coping plan formulation, self-appraisal of risk, etc. Moreover, it remains a logical leap from these findings to the notion that cue reactivity causes relapse (and therefore that cue exposure therapy may prevent relapse), although prospective studies (Abrams et al., 1988; Niaura et al., 1989) take a first step in that direction. Finally, it is noteworthy that several of the studies reviewed above found that the magnitude of cue reactivity appeared to be moderated by individual difference variables such as degree of nicotine dependence, length of nicotine deprivation, and smoker typology (stimulant versus sedative).

Cue Exposure Treatments

There is little research on the treatment of smoking through cue exposure. We were able to find only five treatment outcome experiments and one case study in which cue exposure (or a synonym) was explicitly identified as a component of treatment.

Prior to attempting abstinence, the subject in the case study (Self, 1989)— a light to moderate smoker—self monitored her smoking, mood, and urges to smoke for 2 weeks. These data were then used to identify and rank order seven daily cigarettes that were most strongly cue controlled and that elicited the greatest urges. The subject then worked down the list of cigarettes, systematically extinguishing urges to the associated situations. At the appropriate time for each cigarette, she was instructed to place herself in the identified location, handle the cigarette, light it and take one puff without inhaling, and then rate her urge to smoke. This sequence was repeated 10 times per exposure session, which were held daily, until the urge was substantially reduced. After 64 days, urges had been extinguished for all seven of the targeted situations and the subject had reached complete abstinence. One year after treatment, the subject remained abstinent.

Unfortunately, the five randomized treatment outcome studies of cue exposure have not borne out the promise of the case study. Two of the studies compared cue exposure with aversive rapid smoking treatments. Raw & Russell (1980) assigned 49 smokers to one of three treatments: cue exposure, rapid smoking, and a control treatment of supportive counseling. All subjects received seven 45 minute sessions in groups of four or five subjects. The cue exposure procedure consisted of three or four experiences of lighting a cigarette, sometimes taking a non-inhaled puff and then either holding the lit cigarette or watching it burn in an ashtray. Tea and coffee were also provided as additional cues. The therapist offered cigarettes to subjects and lit cigarettes himself. Also, each day after treatment, subjects were instructed to practice cue exposure three times in a favorite smoking environment. Cue exposure, rapid smoking, and support conditions did not produce significantly different outcomes at the end of treatment, nor at 3, 6 or 12 months follow-up. For example, at 1 year post-treatment, 18% of cue exposure subjects were abstinent, compared to 6% of rapid smoking subjects, and 19% of support group subjects.

In a similar study, Corty & McFall (1984) compared cue exposure (called 'response prevention') to rapid smoking. Thirty smokers received eight sessions of either treatment. During the response prevention sessions subjects carried a pack of their favorite cigarettes while listening to an audio tape of smokers and ex-smokers vividly describing their urge to smoke. Subjects were instructed to imagine these scenes, and to try to maximize their own urge to smoke. Each session included two such trials, with a short break between trials during which subjects carried cigarettes. Between sessions, subjects were to enter the situation described on the tape, and stay in that situation until an urge to smoke arose and died out. Before the final session, subjects carried their cigarettes for 24 hours without smoking and then destroyed them. Treatment outcome was assessed at treatment termination and at 1, 3, and 6 months post-treatment. No significant differences were found between the treatments. However, rapid smoking tended to show the superior outcome. For example, at the 6 month follow-up, only 7% of response prevention subjects were abstinent versus 23% of rapid smoking subjects.

Götestam & Melin (1983) compared imaginal cue exposure (called 'covert extinction') to relaxation training and a waiting list control group, with seven subjects in each condition. Treatment was provided on six consecutive days. Each session of covert extinction training consisted of five trials of imaginal smoking in which subjects were instructed not to imagine any sensations (positive or negative) resulting from the smoking. The rationale was that smoking behavior would be extinguished due to the lack of accompanying reinforcement. No significant differences in outcome were found between the conditions at the 1 month follow-up.

Another study compared three smoking cessation treatments: cue exposure (called 'cue extinction'), self-control training (anticipating and planning for high-risk situations, relaxation training, and self-monitoring or smoking urges), and a combination of the two techniques (Lowe et al., 1980, Study 2). Three weeks of treatment were provided to all 42 subjects in the three treatments. Cue extinction treatment included two components. First, subjects identified their three strongest smoking cues and were instructed to avoid smoking in the presence of these cues for 1 week prior to quitting. The second component was 'focused smoking', in which subjects were asked to smoke a cigarette for 5 minutes while concentrating on only the cigarette and the feelings of smoking. The rationale was that smoking in this manner deprived subjects of the usual reinforcement obtained from the social and environmental concomitants of smoking. Outcome was evaluated at 48 hours, 3 months, and 6 months post-treatment. No significant treatment differences were found on abstinence rates or percent reduction in smoking. However, the combined treatment produced significantly fewer days of abstinence by the 6 month follow-up.

Cue exposure has also been used as a technique to maintain treatment gains. Brandon, Zelman & Baker (1987) provided 57 subjects with 2 weeks of coping skills training and rapid smoking. This treatment was followed by 3 months of one of three maintenance procedures: counseling only, counseling plus puffing, or a non-maintenance control. The counseling-only maintenance group comprised additional coping skills training and self-monitoring, information about cue exposure theory, and systematic assignments for subjects to place themselves in situations associated with smoking while resisting the urge to smoke. The counseling-plus-puffing maintenance condition included the same counseling components plus rapid-puffing trials (similar to rapid smoking except that subjects do not inhale). Rapid puffing was conceptualized as unreinforced exposure to smoking stimuli. Outcome was assessed through 1 year post-treatment. The two maintenance conditions produced nearly identical outcomes. When compared to the non-maintenance control condition, they both appeared to delay relapse during the 3 months of additional meetings, with outcome measures reaching significance at 3 and 4 months post-treatment. Thereafter, however, outcome differences disappeared.

In summary, not one study found cue exposure to be superior to any comparison treatment or control condition. However, these studies have many limitations, the most obvious being low statistical power. Across all five studies, the mean number of smokers in the cue exposure conditions was 15—less than one-third the sample size needed to have adequate power (0.80) for detecting even a medium effect size (Cohen, 1988). Thus, it could be argued that cue exposure was not given a fair test. On the other hand, the direction of the intergroup differences and the effect sizes are not encouraging.

A second difficulty is that several of the studies (e.g. Corty & McFall, 1984; Götestam & Melin, 1983) used cue exposure as the only treatment component. It is probably unrealistic to expect any single technique provided in isolation to be effective in changing such a multidetermined behavior as smoking. The most successful treatments tend to involve multiple components (US Department of Health and Human Services, 1988, p. 500), and it is likely that if cue exposure is to provide any unique benefit, it will be when it is included with other pharmacological and psychosocial interventions. Studies are needed that evaluate cue exposure's contribution to a multicomponent treatment package. Unfortunately, the studies that tested multicomponant treatments (e.g. Brandon, Zelman & Baker, 1987) confounded cue exposure with the other elements of the treatment, and therefore could not evaluate the unique contribution of the technique.

Another obstacle to reaching general conclusions from the reviewed studies is the variety of ways that cue exposure was defined and implemented. Both *in vivo* and imaginal exposure trials were used. The number of trials and length of treatment varied greatly. Some treatments began cue exposure prior to subjects reaching abstinence, whereas others used it as a maintenance tool. Studies also differed in whether actual smoking (with or without inhalation) was included as part of the exposure experience. In some studies components of the exposure treatment may have actually undermined its efficacy (e.g. carrying cigarettes; Corty & McFall, 1984). The relative potencies of these different approaches cannot be evaluated because in no study—with the exception of the case report—was an effort made to verify that any extinction to cues ever occurred. In fact, treatment comparison studies are premature until research identifies the necessary characteristics of an exposure intervention.

DESIGNING CUE EXPOSURE FOR NICOTINE DEPENDENCE

Selecting Exposure Cues

In theory, the efficacy of cue exposure therapy should be influenced by the appropriateness of the exposure cues. The task of cue selection may be an especially complex one where smoking cessation is concerned. This is largely attributable to the fact that smoking is a high-frequency behavior. The pack-a-day smoker self-administers approximately 80 000 doses of nicotine (puffs) per year. To the extent that individual smokers adhere to some sort of daily routine, the potential exists for an overwhelming array of stimuli to become correlated with nicotine delivery to the central nervous system. Given that robust Pavlovian conditioning can accrue in as few as eight trials (e.g. Rescorla, 1988), the challenge of optimal cue selection is patent. Clinicians interested in developing cue exposure interventions for smoking cessation will thus find themselves faced with an immense number of potential exposure stimuli.

Theoretical considerations

Conditioning theory can help pare down the types of cues to be used in an exposure paradigm. For example, modern conditioning theory suggests using the most highly salient cues that are correlated with the unconditioned stimulus (US), and also cues that reliably predict changes in US intensity (e.g. Dickinson, Hall & MacKintosh, 1976; Rescorla & Wagner, 1972).

A special class of CSs and SDs are those that simultaneously provoke temptation and interfere with an individual's ability to cope. No general theoretical account has been offered to assist in identifying these cues. Nonetheless, it is likely that alcohol ingestion, negative affective states, and the presence of other smokers may fit this description. For instance, other smokers might facilitate relapse by cajoling the recently-quit into the resumption of smoking. Alcohol (Steele & Josephs, 1988) and affective arousal (Easterbrook, 1959) tend to constrain attention to the most salient stimuli in the immediate environment. If these highly salient stimuli are related to smoking, as alcohol and negative affect may themselves be, the probability of relapse would be augmented. Because they represent more serious threats to prolonged abstinence than their absolute associative strength would imply, clinicians should pay particular attention to cues that could potentially hamper coping.

Leading cue candidates

The theoretical issues outlined above delimit the class of stimuli that appear ideal for cue exposure. However, the number of smoking-related cues meeting these stricter specifications is still likely to be large. Several considerations may be useful in winnowing the myriad of potential cues. One consideration is the frequency with which clients can be expected to encounter them in the natural environment. The difficulty inherent in manipulating exposure to candidate stimuli is a second important consideration. Finally, sensitivity to individual differences in smoking motivation can contribute to effective cue selection.

Some cues can reasonably be expected to pose problems for the majority of quitting smokers. Smoking paraphernalia, environmental tobacco smoke, and components of the action schema associated with the act of smoking perhaps fall most squarely into this category. The sight, smell, and feel of cigarettes, ashtrays, matches, and the like are highly salient stimuli that are highly correlated with nicotine delivery and that will be difficult, if not impossible for smokers to avoid after cessation. Therefore, any effective cue exposure treatment for smoking will incorporate these cues perforce. However, the sequence of behaviors leading to smoking often begins long before the presence of these proximal smoking cues. In theory, it should be possible to interrupt this sequence by also selecting exposure cues that are more distally related to smoking.

The growing literature devoted to the identification of high-risk smoking relapse situations suggests a number of distal cues that are likely to be problematic for quitting smokers. Social situations, often involving food or alcohol consumption, the presence of others smoking, and negative affect are consistently found to be highly associated with relapse (Baer & Lichtenstein, 1988; Brandon et al., 1990; Shiffman, 1982, 1986). The validity of these relapse data are, however, limited by both the means of collection—retrospective self-report—and the (at best) correlational nature of the research. However, the impact of negative affect identified in these cross-sectional studies is consistent with prospective research also showing that negative affect, including clinical depression, is related to smoking relapse (Zelman et al., 1992; Glassman et al., 1988; Hall et al., 1983), and that negative affect plays an important motivational role in the maintenance of smoking in general (Brandon, 1994).

Negative affect may serve other functions in addition to its Pavlovian role. The data relating negative affect to increased self-administration also suggest that negative affective states may become enmeshed in instrumental associations. Negative affect may act as an SD signaling that smoking behavior will result in maximal negative reinforcement (Pomerleau & Pomerleau, 1984; Zinser et al., 1992).

A separate question is whether smokers should be exposed to the self-administration ritual during cue exposure, as has been done in some studies (Brandon, Zelman & Baker, 1987; Lowe et al., 1980; Raw & Russell, 1980). When instrumental responding occurs in the presence of discriminative stimuli, it is possible that diverse associative linkages are formed. Some, such as response–reinforcer associations, may require that the smoking self-administration ritual be practiced repeatedly without the opportunity for reinforcement. This, in fact, may underlie some of the beneficial effects of procedures such as 'rapid puffing' (Tiffany, Martin & Baker, 1986). However, the benefits of including the self-administration ritual *per se* as part of a cue exposure treatment have not yet been empirically investigated.

Selecting smoking cues idiographically

The arsenal of cues outlined above might be augmented with stimuli selected on a more personalized basis. A convenient way this might be accomplished is by administering patients one of several available self-report instruments developed to assess individual differences in smoking motives (e.g. Horn & Waingrow, 1966; McKennell, 1970; Russell, Peto & Patel, 1974). However, a recent review of these measures revealed that their criterion validity is quite low; on average, the scales account for 3.2% of the variance in actual smoking behavior (Shiffman, 1993). This finding discourages reliance upon such measures for the selection of specific exposure cues. Nonetheless, these 'smoking typology' scales might be fruitful when combined with a larger assessment package in order to make relatively coarse decisions about stimulus classes worthy of further examination.

More idiographic information can be collected by having the client self-monitor his or her smoking for a given period of time in order to identify those situational and temporal cues associated with smoking (cf. Self, 1989). Self-monitoring may be enhanced by recent technological advances. Clients can carry small computers that query them at irregular intervals about various features of the immediate situation and whether or not they are smoking (Paty, Kassel & Shiffman, 1992; Shiffman, 1993). At the end of the monitoring period, the data can be retrieved and the correlates of smoking determined. This procedure has the clear advantage of affording investigators a glimpse at the base rates of occurrence of various cues, independent of their co-occurrence with smoking. This is important because cues that are frequently present in the smokers' environment are likely to coincide with smoking, but may or may not be correlated with smoking (e.g. Paty, Kassel & Shiffman, 1992; Sutton, 1993). In theory, only correlated cues should be used in exposure treatment.

Other Considerations When Using Cue Exposure to Treat Nicotine Dependence

The quantity and variety of cues associated with smoking has some additional treatment implications. Because correlations between smoking-relevant cues and nicotine delivery are liable to be based upon countless pairings, many exposure trials may be necessary to undermine their association. The equivocal results of cue exposure studies with smokers may in part be attributable to the relatively small number of exposure trials they have employed.

Additionally, research on reinstatement and renewal effects in Pavlovian and instrumental conditioning highlights the importance of conducting cue exposure in a variety of contexts, especially those in which the problematic associations have been learned (Bouton, 1988). Because some evidence suggests that the functional definition of 'context' is broad, including things like drug-produced stimuli and affective states (Bouton & Swartzentruber, 1991; Bouton, 1988), and because smoking occurs in such varied contexts, it is clear that complete extinction of all important smoking cues across all meaningful contexts is not feasible. This underscores the importance of constructing multi-component treatment packages for smoking cessation rather than relying exclusively on cue exposure strategies.

An important practical question that has received relatively less theoretical attention concerns the optimal modality for exposure cue presentation. Some investigations of cue exposure treatments for smoking have used smoking-related imagery, either alone or in conjunction with external stimuli, to foment motivational responses (Götestam & Melin, 1993; Corty & McFall, 1984; Self, 1989). There are obvious advantages associated with this sort of strategy. For instance, because a great number of cues may serve to maintain smoking and because extinction does not readily generalize across contexts, cue exposure therapy for smoking cessation might prove unwieldy if *in vivo* exposure is used exclusively. Moreover, imagery may be particularly helpful in the clinical elicitation of negative affective states for exposure (e.g. Lang et al., 1980; Tiffany & Drobes, 1990; Tiffany & Hakenewerth, 1991). Because the potential payoffs of imaginal exposure are large, future research should be designed to address its efficacy.

How Should Therapeutic Progress Be Monitored?

This is a difficult question because we do not know what specific responses need to be extinguished, nor do we know how to assess them. As indicated earlier, smoking cue reactivity has been demonstrated in several domains, but it does not seem that these separate responses always cohere (Tiffany & Hakenewerth, 1991; Niaura et al., 1992). In the absence of empirical work linking the modification of specific responses to smoking cessation outcome, it is difficult to suggest how clinicians should assess their progress.

Because drug-engendered responding is multifaceted, measures capable of capturing the summative impact of diverse drug motivational responses may be more clinically useful than individual responses from any single system. Thus, broad measures such as self-reports of smoking urges and perceived self-efficacy might constitute useful clinical metrics. Each of these measures has met with some success in predicting smoking cessation outcomes (West & Schneider, 1987; Killen et al., 1992; Haaga & Stewart, 1992; Condiotte & Lichtenstein, 1981). One problem with such indices, however, is that they may be too broad or integrative to reflect exposure effects *per se*. Another problem with such measures is that they depend upon declarative knowledge and therefore may not capture important motivational changes of which clients are not aware. Clearly, a major goal of future research in the area of cue exposure is the identification of responses that index important motivational effects of cue exposure and that predict post-treatment functioning.

HOW SHOULD AN INTENSIVE EXPOSURE TREATMENT BE DELIVERED?

While specifics of program delivery will be dictated by specific program attributes, some general aspects of program implementation can be anticipated. First, as noted earlier, it seems wise to plan to deliver the cue exposure therapy as part of a multicomponent intervention rather than a stand-alone treatment. Aside from the theoretical rationale for this, it is likely that most clients will receive such therapies as 4 mg nicotine gum or the nicotine transdermal patch because of the relatively low cost, efficacy, and ease of application of these interventions (Fiore et al., 1992; Tang, Law & Wald, 1994).

While there is considerable evidence that such interventions are beneficial as stand-alone treatments, there is also considerable evidence that their efficacy is enhanced by psychosocial treatments. A recent meta-analysis of 17 placebo-controlled, double-blind nicotine patch clinical trials revealed that nicotine patch treatment produces higher abstinence rates when it is used with relatively intense psychosocial interventions (Fiore et al., 1994). Across active patch subjects in the 17 rated studies, an average of 22.6% of subjects were abstinent if the patch was offered with low intensity psychosocial intervention, whereas 40.1% of subjects were abstinent if the patch was paired with more intense psychosocial treatment. These data suggest a substantial pay-off for intensive psychosocial treatments even in the presence of effective pharmacological interventions.

Because some patients will be able to quit without an intensive intervention such as cue exposure, it makes sense that a stepped-care approach be used (e.g. Lichtenstein & Hollis, 1992; Orleans, 1993). In such an approach, all patients interested in quitting smoking would be exposed to a low-cost, relatively non-intensive cessation intervention such as physician advice to quit, a prescription for nicotine replacement, and a follow-up visit or phone call to monitor the patient's progress and provide maintenance assistance. Smokers failing to quit with this approach could then be offered additional, more intensive treatment. It is unclear when this should be offered—when the smoker has recuperated from a failed quit attempt and is ready to initiate an additional attempt (Prochaska, DiClemente & Norcross, 1992), or shortly after it appears that a smoker is failing in the current attempt. The latter option has the advantage of intervening before the smoker suffers some of the negative consequences of a failed attempt that would hinder further cessation efforts (e.g. lowered self-efficacy). Along these lines, Kenford et al. (1994) recently found that any smoking by clients in the first 2 weeks of treatment was a consistent and powerful predictor of long-term failure. Their data show that it is possible to identify the majority of relapsers relatively early in the treatment process, thus making possible an efficient intra-treatment 'step-up' of potential failures to a more intensive intervention. Of course, more research is needed to determine whether step-up approaches do significantly augment cessation rates, when step-up interventions should be delivered, and where in the step care sequence cue exposure approaches belong to maximize cost-effectiveness.

An alternative to a stepped care approach is to try to match patients with treatments prior to treatment implementation. For instance, there is evidence that supportive counseling is especially effective with smokers who report high levels of negative affect prior to, or early in, the quit attempt. Other smokers appear to be helped more by skill training (Zelman et al., 1992). Unfortunately, matching strategies are unlikely to be successful in the very near future given the dearth of data on aptitude–treatment relations in smoking, the lack of data on the mechanisms of action of smoking exposure therapy, and the absence of compelling theories regarding exposure treatment and the nature of addiction.

Finally, it is worth considering whether there even is a role for intensive smoking cessation treatments, such as those that would incorporate cue exposure. The cost-effectiveness of intensive cessation programs has been questioned because a relatively small proportion of smokers enroll in formal programs, and those who do enroll appear to be less successful than smokers who attempt to quit on their own (Fiore et al., 1990). It might be argued, therefore, that limited health-care funds can be better spent on low-cost interventions such as the nicotine patch and physician advice to quit. What this argument fails to consider is that intensive cessation programs tend to attract atypical smokers—those who smoke more, have a greater history of failed quit attempts, score higher on indices of physical dependence, and have less confidence in their ability to quit (Fiore et al., 1990; Lichtenstein & Hollis, 1992). These are the smokers whom we would least expect to benefit from low-intensity interventions, yet they are probably also the smokers who are most at risk for developing smoking-related illnesses. The cost of intensive programs should be evaluated against the cost of continued smoking in these heavily dependent individuals. The most effective strategy for reducing the long-term costs of smoking may be the stepped care approach mentioned earlier, in which intensive interventions are provided to those smokers for whom earlier, low-cost interventions have been unsuccessful. Much more research is needed on the efficacy and optimal delivery of cue exposure for treating nicotine dependence, however, before we can recommend that it be included among those intensive interventions.

ACKNOWLEDGEMENTS

Preparation of this chapter was supported by Grant #JFRA389 from the American Cancer Society and Grant #92–024GB from the American Heart Association, New York State Affiliate, awarded to Thomas H. Brandon.

REFERENCES

Abrams, D.B., Monti, P.M., Carey, K.B., Pinto, R.P. & Jacobus, S.I. (1988). Reactivity to smoking cues and relapse: two studies of discriminant validity. *Behaviour Research and Therapy*, **26**, 225–233.

Baer, J.S. & Lichtenstein, E. (1988). Classification and prediction of smoking relapse episodes: an exploration of individual differences. *Journal of Consulting and Clinical Psychology*, **56**, 104–110.

Bouton, M.E. (1988). Context and ambiguity in the extinction of emotional learning: implications for exposure therapy. *Behavior Research and Therapy*, **26**, 137–149.

Bouton, M.E. & Swartzentruber, D. (1991). Sources of relapse after extinction in Pavlovian and instrumental learning. *Clinical Psychology Review*, **11**, 123–140.

Brandon, T.H. (1994). Negative affect as motivation to smoke. *Current Directions in Psychological Science*, **3**, 33–37.

Brandon, T.H., Wetter, D.W. & Baker, T.B. (1994). Affect expectancies, urges, and smoking: do they conform to models of drug motivation and relapse? Manuscript under review.

Brandon, T.H., Zelman, D.C. & Baker, T.B. (1987). Effects of maintenance sessions on smoking relapse: delaying the inevitable? *Journal of Consulting and Clinical Psychology*, **55**, 780–782.

Brandon, T.H., Tiffany, S.T., Obremski, K.M. & Baker, T.B. (1990). Postcessation cigarette use: the process of relapse. *Addictive Behaviors*, **15**, 105–114.

Cohen, J. (1988). *Statistical Power Analysis for the Behavioral Sciences*, 2nd edn. Hillsdale, NJ: Erlbaum.

Condiotte, M.M. & Lichtenstein, E. (1981). Self-efficacy and relapse in smoking cessation programs. *Journal of Consulting and Clinical Psychology*, **49**, 648–658.

Corty, E. & McFall, R.M. (1984). Response prevention in the treatment of cigarette smoking. *Addictive Behaviors*, **9**, 405–408.

Dickinson, A., Hall, G. & Mackintosh, N.J. (1976). Surprise and the attenuation of blocking. *Journal of Experimental Psychology: Animal Behavior Processes*, **2**, 213–222.

Easterbrook, J.A. (1959). The effect of emotion on cue utilization and the organization of behavior. *Psychological Review*, **66**, 183–201.

Fiore, M.C., Novotny, T.E., Pierce, J.P., Giovino, G.A., Hatziandreu, E.J., Newcomb, P.A., Surawicz, T.S. & Davis, R.M. (1990). Methods used to quit smoking in the United States: do cessation programs help? *Journal of the American Medical Association*, **263**, 2760–2765.

Fiore, M.C., Jorenby, D.E., Baker, T.B. & Kenford, S.L. (1992). Tobacco dependence and the nicotine patch: clinical guidelines for effective use. *Journal of the American Medical Association*, **268**, 2687–2694.

Fiore, M.C., Smith, S.S., Jorenby, D.E. & Baker, T.B. (1994). The effectiveness of the nicotine patch for smoking cessation: a meta-analysis. *Journal of the American Medical Association*, **271**, 1940–1947.

Glassman, A.H., Stetner, F., Walsh, P., Raizman, S., Fleiss, J.L., Cooper, T.B. & Covey, L.S. (1988). Heavy smokers, smoking cessation, and clonidine: results of a double-blind, randomized trial. *Journal of the American Medical Association*, **259**, 2863–2866.

Götestam, K.G. & Melin, L. (1983). An experimental study of covert extinction on smoking cessation. *Addictive Behaviors*, **8**, 27–31.

Haaga, D.A.F. & Stewart, B.L. (1992). Self-efficacy for recovery from a lapse after smoking cessation. *Journal of Consulting and Clinical Psychology*, **60**, 24–28.

Hall, S.M., Bachman, J., Henderson, J.B., Barstow, R. & Jones, R.T. (1983). Smoking cessation in patients with cardiopulmonary disease: an initial study. *Addictive Behaviors*, **8**, 33–42.

Hall, S.M., Rugg, D., Tunstall, C. & Jones, R.T. (1984). Preventing relapse to cigarette smoking by behavioral skill training. *Journal of Consulting and Clinical Psychology*, **52**, 372–382.

Herman, C.P. (1974). External and internal cues as determinants of the smoking behavior of light and heavy smokers. *Journal of Personality and Social Psychology*, **30**, 664–672.

Horn, D. & Waingrow, S. (1966). Some dimensions of a model for smoking behavior change. *American Journal of Public Health*, **56** (Suppl.), 21–26.

Kenford, S.L., Fiore, M.C., Jorenby, D.E., Smith, S.S., Wetter, D. & Baker, T.B. (1994). Predicting smoking cessation: who will quit with and without the nicotine patch. *Journal of the American Medical Association*, **271**, 589–594.

Killen, J.D., Fortmann, S.P., Kraemer, H.C., Varady, A. & Newman, B. (1992). Who will relapse? Symptoms of nicotine dependence predict long-term relapse after smoking cessation. *Journal of Consulting and Clinical Psychology*, **60**, 797–801.

Lang, P.J., Kozak, M.J., Miller, G.A., Levin, D.N. & McLean, A., Jr (1980). Emotional imagery: conceptual structure and pattern of somatovisceral response. *Psychophysiology*, **17**, 179–192.

Lichtenstein, E. & Hollis, J. (1992). Patient referral to a smoking cessation program: who follows through? *Journal of Family Practice*, **34**, 739–744.

Lowe, M.R., Green, L., Kurtz, S.M.S., Ashenberg, Z.S. & Fisher, E.B.,Jr (1980). Self-initiated, cue-extinction, and covert sensitization procedures in smoking cessation. *Journal of Behavioral Medicine*, **3**, 357–372.

McKennel, A.C. (1970). Smoking motivation factors. *British Journal of Social and Clinical Psychology*, **9**, 8–22.

Niaura, R., Abrams, D.B., Monti, P.M. & Pedraza, M. (1989). Reactivity to high risk situations and smoking cessation outcome. *Journal of Substance Abuse*, **1**, 393–405.

Niaura, R., Abrams, D.B., Pedraza, M., Monti, P.M. & Rohsenow, D.J. (1992). Smokers' reactions to interpersonal interaction and presentation of smoking cues. *Addictive Behaviors*, **17**, 557–566.

Orleans, T.C. (1993). Treating nicotine dependence in medical settings: a stepped-care model. In C.T. Orleans & J. Slade (Eds), *Nicotine Addiction: Principles and Management*, pp. 145–161. New York: Oxford University Press.

Paty, J., Kassel, J. & Shiffman, S. (1992). Assessing stimulus control of smoking: the importance of base rates. In M. DeVries (Ed.), *The Experience of Psychopathology*, pp. 347–352. Cambridge: Cambridge University Press.

Payne, T.J., Etscheidt, M. & Corrigan, S.A. (1990). Conditioning arbitrary stimuli to cigarette smoke intake: a preliminary study. *Journal of Substance Abuse*, **2**, 113–119.

Payne, T.J., Schare, M.L., Levis, D.J. & Colletti, G. (1991). Exposure to smoking-relevant cues: effects on desire to smoke and topographical components of smoking behavior. *Addictive Behaviors*, **16**, 467–479.

Pomerleau, O.F. & Pomerleau, C.S. (1984). Neuroregulators and the reinforcement of smoking behavior: towards a biobehavioral explanation. *Neuroscience and Biobehavioral Reviews*, **8**, 503–513.

Prochaska, J.O., DiClemente, C.C. & Norcross, J. (1992). In search of how people change: applications to addictive behavior. *American Psychologist*, **47**, 1102–1114.

Raw, M. & Russell, M.A.H. (1980). Rapid smoking, cue exposure, and support in the modification of smoking. *Behavior Research and Therapy*, **18**, 363–372.

Rescorla, R.A. (1988). Ravlovian conditioning: it's not what you think it is. *American Psychologist*, **43**, 151–160.

Rescorla, R.A. & Wagner, A.R. (1972). A theory of Pavlovian conditioning: variations in the effectiveness of reinforcement and nonreinforcement. In A.H. Black & W.F. Prokasy (Eds), *Classical Conditioning II: Current Theory and Research*, pp. 64–99. New York: Appleton-Century-Crofts.

Rickard-Figueroa, K. & Zeichner, A. (1985). Assessment of smoking urge and its concomitants under an environmental smoking cue manipulation. *Addictive Behaviors*, **10**, 249–256.

Russell, M.A.H., Peto, J. & Patel, U.A. (1974). The classification of smoking by factorial structure of motives. *Journal of the Royal Statistical Society*, **137**, 313–346.

Sayette, M.A. & Hufford, M.R. (1993). Cognitive effects of cue exposure in smokers. Paper presented at the meeting of the Association for Advancement of Behavior Therapy, Atlanta.

Sayette, M.A. & Hufford, M.R. (1994). Effects of cue exposure and deprivation on cognitive resources in smokers. *Journal of Abnormal Psychology*, **103**, 812–818.

Self, R. (1989). The effect of cue-exposure response prevention on cigarette smoking—a single case. *Behavioural Psychotherapy*, **17**, 151–159.

Shiffman, S. (1982). Relapse following smoking cessation: a situational analysis. *Journal of Consulting and Clinical Psychology*, **50**, 71–86.

Shiffman, S. (1986). A cluster-analytic classification of smoking relapse episodes. *Addictive Behaviors*, **11**, 295–307.

Shiffman, S. (1993). Assessing smoking patterns and motives. *Journal of Comparative and Clinical Psychology*, **61**, 732–742.

Steele, C.M. & Josephs, R.A. (1988). Drinking your troubles away II: an attention-allocation model of alcohol's effects on psychological stress. *Journal of Abnormal Psychology*, **97**, 196–205.

Surawy, C., Stepney, R. & Cox, T. (1985). Does watching others smoke increase smoking? *British Journal of Addiction*, **80**, 207–210.

Sutton, S. (1993). Is wearing clothes a high-risk situation for relapse? The base rate problem in relapse research. *Addiction*, **88**, 725–727.

Tang, J.L., Law, M. & Wald, N. (1994). How effective is nicotine replacement therapy in helping people to stop smoking? *Lancet*, **308**, 21–26.

Tiffany, S.T. & Drobes, D.J. (1990). Imagery and smoking urges: the manipulation of affective content. *Addictive Behaviors*, **15**, 531–539.

Tiffany, S.T. & Hakenewerth, D.M. (1991). The production of smoking urges through an imagery manipulation: Psychophysiological and verbal manifestations. *Addictive Behaviors*, **16**, 389–400.

Tiffany, S.T., Martin, E.M. & Baker, T.B. (1986). Treatments for cigarette smoking: an evaluation of the contributions of aversion and counseling procedures. *Behaviour Research and Therapy*, **24**, 437–452.

US Department of Health and Human Services (1988). *The Health Consequences of Smoking: Nicotine Addiction. A Report of the Surgeon General*. Washington, DC: US Government Printing Office.

West, R.J. & Schneider, N. (1987). Craving for cigarettes. *British Journal of Addiction*, **82**, 407–415.

Zelman, D.C., Brandon, T.H., Jorenby, D.E. & Baker, T.B. (1992). Measures of affect and nicotine dependence predict differential response to smoking cessation. *Journal of Consulting and Clinical Psychology*, **60**, 943–952.

Zinser, M.C., Baker, T.B., Sherman, J.E. & Cannon, D.S. (1992). Relation between self-reported affect and drug urges and cravings in continuing and withdrawing smokers. *Journal of Abnormal Psychology*, **101**, 617–629.

AUTHOR INDEX

SUBJECT INDEX

THE WILEY SERIES IN
CLINICAL PSYCHOLOGY

Roger Baker (Editor)	Panic Disorder: Theory, Research and Therapy
Friedrich Fösterling	Attribution Theory in Clinical Psychology
Anthony Lavender and Frank Holloway (Editors)	Community Care in Practice: Services for the Continuing Care Client
J. Mark G. Williams, Fraser N. Watts, Colin MacLeod and Andrew Mathews	Cognitive Psychology and Emotional Disorders
John Clements	Severe Learning Disability and Psychological Handicap

Treatment Approaches for Alcohol and Drug Dependence
An Introductory Guide

TRACEY J. JARVIS, JENNY TEBBUTT and
RICHARD P. MATTICK, *National Drug and Alcohol Research Centre, University of New South Wales, Australia*

A step-by-step guide to applying skills-based therapies to clients with alcohol or other drug dependence/misuse. The authors include case studies to illustrate how the various techniques can be combined and tailored for individual needs, and have also included lists of resources and self-help material which the counsellor may share with their client.

0-471-95373-3   228pp   Paperback   1995

Young Offenders and Alcohol-Related Crime
A Practitioner's Guidebook

MARY MCMURRAN, *Rampton Hospital, Nottingham, UK* and
CLIVE R. HOLLIN, *University of Birmingham, UK*

• **What works with young offenders - particularly those whose crimes were alcohol related?**

This practical guidebook offers a framework for the development of a cognitive-behavioural programme with young offenders. The programme deals with the different stages of intervention from screening for problems through to encouraging positive changes in lifestyle.

0-471-93839-4   208pp   Paperback   1993

Excessive Appetites
A Psychological View of Addictions

JIM ORFORD, *University of Birmingham, UK*

"... a valuable addition to the literature... it presents a lucid and highly informative account of the major issues in addictions. It can be highly recommended."

BRITISH JOURNAL OF ADDICTION

0-471-93613 8   378pp   Paperback   1992